When Blushing Hurts

When Blushing Hurts

Overcoming Abnormal Facial Blushing

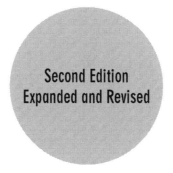

Second Edition
Expanded and Revised

Enrique Jadresic, MD

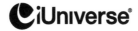

WHEN BLUSHING HURTS
OVERCOMING ABNORMAL FACIAL BLUSHING

iUniverse Star
an iUniverse LLC imprint

iUniverse books may be ordered through booksellers or by contacting:

iUniverse
1663 Liberty Drive
Bloomington, IN 47403
www.iuniverse.com
1-800-Authors (1-800-288-4677)

ISBN: 978-1-5320-2054-4 (sc)
ISBN: 978-1-5320-2053-7 (e)

Library of Congress Control Number: 2014918577

Print information available on the last page.

iUniverse rev. date: 03/30/2017

To those who are hurting and are too embarrassed to reach out for help.

Blushing is the most peculiar and the most human of all expressions.

—Charles Darwin

Man is the only animal that blushes. Or needs to.

—Mark Twain

Contents

Part One
Personal/Medical Itinerary

Part Two
The Light at the End of the Tunnel

Foreword to the First Edition (2008)

Reading a book such as *When Blushing Hurts* gives rise to a multitude of reflections, questions, and approaches that go beyond the perusal of an eminently instructive text or a collection of clinical cases, characteristics that can clearly be assigned, of course, to this volume. When I consider the reason for this fascinating difference, the answer returns loud and clear: At the heart of the book is a personal testimony; an intense, decisive clinical experience; and a *princeps* case told with courage, genuine sensitivity, empathy, and honesty. This reason alone is enough to justify the attention given to it, but, fortunately for the readers, the book offers much more. It undoubtedly has the merit of shedding new light on a clinical disorder that is much more common than we can imagine; it also presents vital syndromic, nosologic, and therapeutic concepts as well as a universal call for an unprejudiced, objective, and holistic look at people who suffer, often in silence, from the dramatic ambiguity of "the most human of all expressions."

The wealth of clinical, scientific, and technical information in the book is extraordinary. The distinction made between "basic" and "higher" emotions vis-à-vis blushing is precise and pertinent. The comment that "It is incorrect to associate blushing only with fear or anxiety ..." opens up a thoughtful debate on adaptive responses, emotional expressiveness, neuropsychological sequences (and the reverse), and diagnostic criteria. For the latter field, the phenomenological description of the author presiding over a class meeting at school is revealing, and admirably so. The reflections and questions that succeeded the experience: the sequence of symptoms, irrational fear, expectations, perceptions, comments, and third-party interpretations; these are all valid and consistent. The questions that arise concerning differences in intergenerational attitudes toward blushing are also relevant.

The discussion of whether pathological blushing (PB) is an illness is a timely one in view of current and future debates on diagnostic and classification systems in psychiatry. Dr. Jadresic's answer is clear: PB must be considered a morbid symptom or a psychiatric disorder when it is triggered by "minor psychological precipitants, causes psychological suffering, and interferes significantly with a person's academic/occupational functioning or interpersonal relations." Citing Edelmann, one of the few authors who have addressed the subject, he establishes needed clinical distinctions which provide the basis for differential diagnoses that, in the nosological context, are also crucial.

The chapter on therapeutic options is essential to the structure and purposes of the book. Drug therapy and cognitive-behavioral techniques are cited first, clearly a justified approach for treating both PB and SAD, a related disorder. The combined use of these methods is an equally valid alternative. The greatest and most novel emphasis, however, is on the endoscopic thoracic sympathectomy (ETS), a procedure that has existed for quite some time but has undeniably been perfected through modern technology. The author's own case and various others included in the rich collection of the second part of the book are valuable contributions to the literature on the topic. Each case (documented with measurement scales and personal testimonies) offers a unique perspective and experience: from the grim reality of social ostracism to the joy of personal "rediscovery," from deep depression and intense self-reproach to the decision to "learn to live again," from the exploration of an enigmatic "family incidence" to the "radical change in personality" resulting from the treatment. The ethnographic character of these stories and the human warmth expressed in sincere gratitude give this book a deeper dimension. The opening quotes and the chapter notes are worthwhile additions: the former, telling; the latter, informative. Moreover, it should be understood that, to the best of our knowledge, this is the first book on the subject written by a psychiatrist, one more distinction that does justice to the quality, vision, and talents of its author.

I have known Enrique Jadresic for many years. I am familiar with his illustrious intellectual heritage, I know of his brilliant professional background, I appreciate his contributions to Chilean and Spanish-language psychiatry and medicine, and I have witnessed his excellence in teaching. Despite the distance separating us, both in geography and in time, I am bound to him and to many other colleagues in Chile through a friendship that is more of an intense, warm brotherhood, reaffirmed by our common interest in the area we chose as the vital spark of our professional activity. While reading *When Blushing Hurts*, I once again admired his expository talent; his elegant, poetic pen; his thoughtful honesty; and his clinical ability. I join with him in calling on psychiatrists and health-care professionals to participate actively in the study of this and other clinical disorders, to approach issues of controversy and debate with both passion and objectivity, to explore the transcultural applicability of all clinical phenomena, to promote investigation, and to improve the level of information available to the general public on the clinical realities that we as physicians confront day after day. Enrique says in his book that emotions are an essential ingredient to the individual identity. From this it could be inferred that if a person's emotional life is rich and sensitive, the identity of that person will be vital and solid, and fully human. Because, as Anatole Broyard said, "a doctor, like a writer, must have a voice of his own, something that conveys the timbre, the rhythm, the diction, and the music of his humanity …" Enrique Jadresic has done just that.

Renato D. Alarcón, MD, MPH
Professor of Psychiatry
Mayo Medical School
Rochester, Minnesota

Prologue to the Second Edition (2014)

It was in 2003 that I first had patients coming to me seeking relief from blushing. By 2007, when I wrote the first edition of this book, I had seen roughly 150 patients. It may not seem like many, but it was quite a large number for any doctor at that time, because people who suffered from debilitating facial blushing tended not to seek help, either simply because they did not know that help was available or because they did not dare come forward to ask. In other words, although blushing was a well-known phenomenon, most laypeople and health professionals were not aware that blushing could become a relevant clinical symptom and could even at times be disabling.

Back then, almost no one who arrived at my office sought me out directly, but they did so at the recommendation of a thoracic surgeon. The publication of *When Blushing Hurts* is undoubtedly what was most instrumental in changing that situation. Nowadays, most patients seek me out spontaneously, many of them telling me that I am the first person they have ever confided in since, out of embarrassment, they have not even shared their struggles with those they are closest to.

Over the last decade, I have met with more than seven hundred patients for their difficulties with blushing. I have also been in remote contact—through e-mail, Skype, and the social networks—with people from many different countries, mostly in Latin America but also in Spain, the United States, England, Poland, and South Korea. This list reflects the prevalence of a condition that, even just a few years ago, the medical world did not address adequately, and for me personally, it has meant an enriched clinical experience that has provided me with opportunities for reflection and learning.

In this second edition of the book, along with sharing new testimonies of women and men who have sought help for blushing, I have whenever possible updated the stories of patients whose cases were told in the first edition. I hope this approach will satisfy those readers who have expressed to me their desire to know the current situation of those people, while, at the same time, I adhere to the medical practice of carrying out a long-term clinical follow-up on the patients who consult us, especially when we are dealing with pathologies that we do not yet fully understand.

Finally, I am happy to say that there has been a significant increase in recent years in the number of scientific papers and publications on blushing. The work in this area has been done from very different perspectives, all of them valuable and complementary. The purpose of this new edition is to update our understanding on those who seek medical help for blushing in light of this new knowledge. While this book is aimed primarily at people who struggle with blushing, I also hope to introduce their family members as well as health professionals and interested readers to this exciting new field.

Enrique Jadresic
Santiago
November 2014

Acknowledgments

In the remote land of Chile, my native country, I was lucky enough to be contacted by a number of patients seeking relief for their uncontrollable facial blushing. What they shared with me sparked my interest and intellectual curiosity, but it also touched me deep inside: I felt identified and moved. If I have decided to tell some of their stories, it is because I believe that doing so can help other people all over the world who unknowingly, in silence and loneliness, suffer from the same affliction. I am deeply indebted to these patients, who trusted in me and gave me permission to use their testimonies as a major portion of this book. I am grateful to them not only for their generosity in agreeing to share their experiences with others but also for the creative resonance of their words. Their accounts motivated me to tell fragments of my own story, which is similar to theirs in many respects.

I would also like to thank Dr. Claudio Suárez, my own physician, who put me in contact with the protagonists of these stories, and Dr. Estela Palacios, who was a great help in researching the disorder that affects these patients.

Part One

Personal/Medical Itinerary

Introduction

I would not have imagined it possible for such patients to exist; or, if they existed, to remain undescribed. For physicians do not go to, and reports do not emerge, from the "lower reaches," these abysses of affliction, which are now (so to speak) beneath the notice of Medicine.

—Oliver Sacks

Many people will be surprised by this book. On the one hand, very little has been written on the subject of blushing, and on the other, most people assume that facial reddening is simply a natural human reaction to certain situations. But is this really the case? Mightn't the most human of expressions become a torment? I will attempt to show that sometimes blushing is a source of suffering and can, in cases that warrant it, be treated.

I would like to make it clear from the start that I am not referring to the mere fear of blushing, or *erythrophobia*, without facial reddening visible to the naked eye, but to sudden facial reddening that is easily visible to others. As we will see in chapters 1 and 3, blushing in interpersonal encounters is normal if it occurs in proportion to the situation causing it, does not produce psychological suffering to the individual, and does not interfere with the subject's normal life. However, I consider it abnormal if it occurs as a response to minor psychological signs or for no apparent reason, if it causes the person to suffer, and if it interferes with his or her usual level of performance and/or social interactions. Certainly, when blushing is of the latter type, erythrophobia occurs as a matter of course.

I will turn to memory, that ability to take in information, store it, and refer back to it when necessary. I will call on what I have experienced

1

personally and what I have learned through my patients' experiences, all of which has helped me to build and nurture my own identity, while at the same time to define that of others. In medicine, and above all in psychiatry, describing the present in terms of the past rather than in the now or the future opens up a fertile area for exploring and identifying a person's psychological profile. Also, accompanying patients, with empathy,[1] back into their biographical experiences relies heavily on memory, and it is as enriching for the person reaching out for help as for the one attempting to provide it.

Of course, what frequently happens to doctors who write is that when we want to put down on paper the landscapes accessed by our memories, we find that we must choose one of two paths: the concise and strict, but cold, language of the scientist, or the more subjective and personal expression of the individual. Certainly, our professional activities push us more toward the former because from our student days we have been taught to avoid falling into the use of the subjective, the emotional. Consequently, while I would like the spirit of this book to be warm and congenial rather than simply to state scientific findings, I suspect that, to some extent, the physician's predominant tendency to be objective and to speak to the intellect will sometimes come to the fore. At the same time, my role as university professor may at times give my writing an academic bent. In all, I would like to emphasize that the two possible paths, while completely different, are—as all opposites are—complementary; they are not mutually exclusive but rather mutually nourishing. The same thing occurs with a doctor treating his or her patients: we are better professionals when we place as much emphasis on feelings and compassion as we do on scientific precision.

That being said, I would also like to state that, above all, my purpose is to help people, mostly teens and young adults, who suffer from their

---

1 The word *empathy* is derived from the Greek *em* (in) and *pathos* (feeling). The term refers to the emotional process through which we enter the inner world of another person and therefore experience that world indirectly. Psychiatrist Sydney Bloch has said that empathy is a quality essential to anyone attempting to heal. He suggests that, in order to achieve an empathetic and compassionate attitude toward patients and their families, it is necessary to consider the human and scientific aspects as equally important and complementary. See S. Bloch (2005).

propensity to blush easily. While the precise frequency of pathological blushing (PB) remains unknown, current studies suggest that between 5 and 7 percent of the population suffers from this disorder (see chapter 3).

How I wish books like this one had existed when I was an adolescent, one with true stories with which people could identify! To be true to my goal of creating such a book, I have had to overcome my natural reticence and reserve and share aspects of my own "case" as well, convinced that I have no alternative if my desire is for my words to transmit not only the knowledge I have gleaned as a medical doctor but also the emotional experience I have had as both professional and patient.

Anyone who has been in the medical profession in the past few decades has seen the notable advances made in medicine and technology and has confirmed almost daily that our therapeutic resources have increased and improved. This is a well-known fact and one that is discussed regularly in the media. At the same time, however, clinical doctors perceive other changes that do not receive nearly as much attention. One of these changes is indisputably the positive impact the Internet has had on the amount of information available to our patients, although obviously the information is not always reliable and well balanced.

I would like to highlight a few facts regarding the problems that frequent or excessive facial blushing can cause in people's lives, as well as possible treatments, which are the topics covered in this book.

The first is that, precisely because of blushing, it is very difficult to admit that one suffers from blushing. I remember the case of a patient who suffered from severe blushing and was going to undergo surgery to treat it, but she could not summon up the courage to tell her husband. Since she knew that the surgery was also an effective treatment for hyperhidrosis, which was not her diagnosis but one that it was easier for her to "admit" to, she started on a "campaign" to convince her husband that she suffered from excessive perspiring to such a degree that it required surgery. She began to complain that she was perspiring a lot, that it was hot, etc. Clearly, the situation called for a brief but timely round of psychotherapy that relieved the patient's anxiety and enabled her not only to tell her husband the real reason for the surgery but to gain his full support as well. I also remember other cases: the patient who dared tell his partner that his blushing was causing him problems only once he was sure that the place they would meet would be quite dark, or the one who took his mother for a ride in the car when he decided to tell her in order to avoid looking her in the eyes. We generally think that people blush when they are embarrassed. Rarely do we consider the opposite situation: that blushing can cause embarrassment.

Next, I would like to point out that most of my patients come to me after conducting Internet searches. Undoubtedly, the World Wide Web has become a source of readily accessible information where people can research complaints about which, many times, they hesitate to ask their doctors. I am glad of this, but, of course, I also wish these people felt comfortable and accepted enough by their doctors to share these intimate psychological matters with them.

When the first version of *When Blushing Hurts* was published, there were almost no books on the market exclusively on facial blushing. The only exceptions were perhaps two books written by psychologists: One groundbreaking text, which is frequently quoted, is by Robert Edelmann, but it barely touches on pharmacological treatments, much less surgery.[2] Another well-documented but accessible work is by W. Ray Crozier.[3] In addition, W. Ray Crozier and Peter J. Wong recently published a worthwhile, and very complete, reference work that compiles the contributions of the field's most renowned researchers.[4]

Initially, then, I felt compelled to write this book since I had for some time found myself, quite unexpectedly, working in the study of pathological blushing and its possible treatments, a field of medicine known to very few people. Even fewer people had experienced the condition from two standpoints: first as patient and then as a physician treating people suffering from the same condition. Sharing my testimony therefore seemed not just a personal challenge but a kind of ethical imperative, all the more so considering my conviction that the information here can be applied cross-culturally and can potentially help people in places as varied as Manchester, Yokohama, and the southern tip of South America.

Given the nature of this book, I have changed the names of my patients, their locales, and other circumstantial details. However, since their written

---

2 See R. J. Edelmann (1990/2004).
3 See W. R. Crozier (2006).
4 See W. R. Crozier and P. J. de Jong (2013).

or oral accounts have a life of their own, I have attempted to leave them unchanged both in retelling and in adding my own observations.

Finally, as those who have read the first edition will note, this second version shows that helping people who seek medical treatment for blushing is more complex than may have been suggested in the first edition, and it adds different nuances and emphases. Nevertheless, I believe that the book's underlying purpose, as well as its message of hope, remains unchanged.

Chapter 1
Discovering the Emotions

Man, rather than a reasoning animal, is a feeling animal.
—Miguel de Unamuno

In my case, the first unpleasant memories of my own propensity to blush go back to the years of puberty and adolescence. I could recount various episodes, but I will mention one that comes easily to mind. As vice president of my class, I was presiding over a meeting of my class at school in the absence of the president. As the meeting went on and for reasons that I have now forgotten, I suddenly felt my cheeks begin to burn, which automatically caused me to feel intensely embarrassed; this reaction probably only increased the reddening, starting a vicious cycle of blushing and anxiety. Despite the mental and even physical awkwardness that almost invariably, to some degree, affects those who blush, I had the presence of mind to tell my homeroom teacher that I felt ill and was going to the restroom for a moment.

"But, Jadresic," she protested, "you are presiding over the session! You can't just walk out on the class!"

But it was no use. The distress brought on by the waves of color washing over my face made me dash out of the classroom in an effort to calm the red in my cheeks, leaving my teacher nonplussed but resigned. I have the feeling that the "halo effect,"[5] which works to the benefit of

---

5 The halo effect is a cognitive bias leading one to believe that limited attributes can be applied to the whole. For example, if a child is cute, we tend to assume he or she is more

those who enjoy a good reputation—the Jadresic brothers were known for being good students—saved me, since the teacher kept my classmates under control while I was out of the room. I went to the restroom, splashed water on my face, and returned somewhat more poised to the classroom.

In retrospect, and in keeping with previous considerations, it is important to note that the presence of others—my classmates—was a crucial element in the negative connotation the experience took on for me. Certainly, what disturbed me was not the blushing itself or the possibility that it might be an indication of a disorder of some kind. Up until that time, I had never been bothered by the scrutiny of others. My irrational fear had to do with the humiliation and shame that were associated with the unexpected episode of blushing I was experiencing. As I write this decades later, I find it interesting to reflect on the fact that I am sure I would not have felt distressed if I had turned crimson and perspired while alone. It is paradoxical, I think, that the human is such a gregarious animal while, at the same time, the presence of others can be so intimidating.

Despite the fact that this was a crucial episode in my life, I told my parents nothing of my unpleasant experience. Perhaps it was not in character for me to share it, or maybe it was because parents at that time tended to remain more distant from their children. As a result, the adolescents of my generation did not feel close enough to our parents to share our problems with them, at least not in my environment while I was growing up. In addition, I would venture to say that back then we tended not to share our most private emotions with other adults either (mental health professionals, for example) and that, in general, society did not encourage opportunities for opening up emotionally.[6]

---

intelligent. Likewise, if we know that someone is under psychiatric treatment, we tend to see indications of mental illness even in that person's normal, simple actions. The halo effect consists of a generalization based on a specific characteristic, even when the person's other traits do not point in the same direction.

6 In this regard, I believe that the introduction of the concept of *emotional intelligence*, a term coined by two Yale University psychologists (Meter Salovey and John Mayer) and made popular throughout the world by the psychologist and writer Daniel Goleman, has made a major contribution to psychological culture in general. Emotional intelligence refers to the capacity to feel, understand, control, and modify one's own and others' moods. Given the emphasis our world places on intelligence, the term has had the merit of conferring importance on talents such as empathy that previously went unrecognized.

The episode must certainly have left its mark on me, acting as a kind of negative reinforcement that led me to shun attention in order to prevent the onset of anxiety. In fact, the episodes of blushing did recur, and I developed a new desire to remain unnoticed. Still, I would occasionally feel a strong urge to speak out in the presence of others, believing at times that I truly did have something worthwhile to share. On the last day of school before graduation, at the end of 1973, I found myself struggling with an overwhelming ambivalence. On the one hand, I was dying to say something in front of my classmates and our homeroom teacher, and on the other, I was terrified at the prospect of another episode of blushing. Finally, not without first experiencing that gut-wrenching dread so typical of intense anxiety, I was able to speak coherently in front of the class. I must confess, however, that in order to work up my courage and overcome my self-imposed isolation, I first drank, almost instinctively, a little mint liqueur, the first alcoholic beverage I found and surreptitiously slipped from my father's liquor cabinet. Hours later, it gave me great satisfaction to know that I had dared to address my classmates, especially at a time when, in my country, soccer matches and the heavily attended political meetings were almost the only stages (other than romantic conquests, naturally) on which young people had a chance to "perform" in public. Therefore, speaking in public provided an opportunity to confirm one's identity. Still, I was aware that having turned to alcohol, a fact that only one of my classmates discovered (and confronted me with), cast a shadow over my achievement.

Perhaps because I am the son of a psychiatrist and a psychology specialist (my mother's field is the psychology of art), I became aware at a very young age that emotions are inextricably woven into the fabric of human life. Then, when I was thirteen or fourteen, I read that an emotion is an indissoluble feeling made up of various aspects. It is a psychological experience, a physiological event with physical symptoms (including palpitations, sweating, shaking, dry mouth, stomach upset, muscle tension, blushing, or paling), and, simultaneously, a behavior. I discovered for myself that this was true as I observed my own reactions to different situations.

A scene from a book I read recently illustrates the physiological and behavioral aspects I have mentioned as well as an overall characteristic of emotion and of blushing in particular: its treacherous uncontrollability. In the book, Julius, a group therapy leader, immediately sees the automatic overreaction of a part of one patient's nervous system; the scene illustrates how an emotion betrays the one experiencing it, while at the same time demonstrating what health professionals know—that it is anchored in the body:

"Philip remained silent and shook his head slightly [nonverbal behavior]. But his face, now flushed [physiological aspect], said volumes. Julius noted to himself that Philip had a functioning autonomic nervous system after all [anatomical substrate of the emotion]".[7]

We must keep in mind that emotions, one of the essential ingredients of the individual identity, express themselves in different ways. To be precise, most neuroscience experts today recognize six basic emotions: anger, disgust, fear, joy, sadness, and surprise. Studies done in different parts of the world have shown that the facial expressions associated with these emotions are universal and are genetically based. Moreover, animals experience many of the emotions that humans do, such as fear, for example; this is a fact that no zoologist would question today and that most ordinary people accept as natural.

There are also other emotions that, for lack of a better term, have been called higher, or secondary, emotions. While this range of emotions has not been defined as fully as the more basic ones, these include such experiences as guilt, embarrassment, shame, and affection. Several of these emotions depend in part on what the person experiencing them thinks about others, but they also hinge on what that person believes others are thinking about him or her. For example, embarrassment is an unpleasant emotional state that we experience when we know that we have been caught in an individual act or condition that is socially or professionally unacceptable. Embarrassment is similar to shame, except that we can feel ashamed of something that we alone know about ourselves, while embarrassment requires the presence of another person.[8] In addition, embarrassment is

---

7 This novel, *The Schopenhauer Cure*, is a best seller about group psychotherapy narrated by a psychotherapist named Julius Hertzfeld. The book was written by the well-known existentialist psychiatrist and psychotherapist Irvin D. Yalom. See I. D. Yalom (2005).
8 However, there are descriptions of, and I have interviewed, people who have reported blushing in private. When this occurs, the situations they describe are interpersonal

generally understood to be brought on by an action that is merely socially unacceptable rather than one that is morally reprehensible. Blushing, of course, falls into the category of higher, or secondary, emotions. It is incorrect to associate blushing with only fear or anxiety, both of which are primary emotions, since, despite being related to the autonomic nervous system, blushing is different. While anxiety is a more basic emotion, facial reddening, as we shall see, is associated primarily with self-conscious emotions, such as embarrassment, shame, or guilt. The function of these more complex emotions, according to some researchers, is to motivate us to adhere to social norms.[9]

We should note here that emotions are inherent to the human experience and that—when they are normal—they promote an appropriate adaptive response to situations of tension, danger, or threat. Moreover, many people believe that there are no negative emotions and that only two factors can make them potentially negative: their duration and cognitions, which are the thoughts that accompany the emotions. Following this logic, anger, within certain limits, is a useful reaction when we feel our territory is threatened, sadness can help us to heal ourselves through introspection, fear protects us from the dangers around us, and guilt allows us to redeem ourselves. Blushing, analogously, can fulfill a social function, serving as a means of communication. This observation leads us immediately to the need to differentiate blushing as a subjective experience from blushing as a signal; that is, as a message to others of the same species. Empirical evidence supports the hypothesis that the facial reddening that accompanies embarrassment may soften a negative evaluation from those around us. Studies have been carried out in which subjects are shown a series of short scenes involving minor public disturbances, such as someone knocking over a stack of cans in a supermarket. The actor in the first film blushes; the one in the second looks around, embarrassed; and in the third film the actor walks out of the store with no reaction whatsoever.

---

despite the fact that they are alone. Several patients have described blushing while talking on the telephone (or, for example, while receiving an obscene phone call). These are cases of people who, despite being physically alone, are experiencing an interpersonal encounter and, besides, are exposed to a social situation that they did not seek out and that they find unpleasant.

9 See D. Keltner (2003).

When the subjects watching the tapes were asked to judge the situations, they considered the situations to be less serious when the actor blushed or looked embarrassed. The actor that blushed was considered the least guilty of the three and was evaluated more positively than the ones who looked embarrassed or left the supermarket as if nothing had happened. The one who reddened was perceived as more trustworthy, friendly, and deserving of affection than the one who simply looked embarrassed.[10]

However, our concern here is for blushing that is disproportionate to the situation causing it or that occurs for no apparent reason; in other words, on facial reddening that is experienced as something alien that invades the individual, is perceived as a disturbing psychological experience lacking in "legitimacy," as it were, and that causes emotional pain.

In the field of medicine, it is interesting to note that today's neuroimaging techniques show that all the emotions mentioned above, both the higher and the primary, are located in specific neuronal circuits that can be pinpointed through sophisticated medical technologies, including functional magnetic resonance imaging.[11]

Let's turn again to my own experiences with emotions. Later, as I entered the university, things were no easier for me. I had graduated from a public high school, Boys' School No. 8, which had provided me with an education that was markedly deficient when compared to that of my classmates, most of whom were graduates of private prep schools. Also, I had entered medical school with a high-visibility surname, especially in the medical world. An uncle of mine, my father's brother, had been the dean of the school of medicine at the University of Chile and candidate for rector of the same university, and my parents both worked in the same hospital where I was studying. It was not unusual, then, to hear my professors saying such things as "Let's see, who's Jadresic?" on the first day of classes.

It was natural for the professors, several of whom knew of or were acquainted with my parents, to wonder who the young Jadresic was, totally unaware of the effect it had on me. I suffered waves of anxiety every time attendance was called in class or when a student might be called on,

---

10 See P. J. de Jong (1999).
11 Functional magnetic resonance imaging (FMRI) is a clinical and research procedure that presents images showing the areas of the brain that perform a specific task. No injections of any substances are required for an FMRI.

believing my chances for being singled out were high and dreading an episode of blushing. By this time, I was clearly suffering from a fear of blushing in public, known as *erythrophobia*, or *ereuthrophobia*. The worst thing was having my peers confirm that I did indeed redden frequently and that there was absolutely nothing I could do about it.

Many people will wonder if I am not simply being egocentric and exaggerating the situation. I do not think so. All genuine pain, whether physical or emotional, is ultimately subjective and self-centered. This was a very unpleasant, egodystonic[12] experience for me, one in which I felt strange, foreign, even alien to myself and my most basic nature, as I was outgoing and eager for friends, which I believed I did indeed have. Besides, it was something beyond my control. It kept me from being the master of my own body, and as it recurred, time and again, it began slowly but surely, and very effectively, to erode my feelings of self-worth.

Other people's expectations of me were a major concern at that time of my life. My twin brother, to the entire family's surprise, earned the highest score in the country on that year's college entrance exam. One hundred thirty thousand students from all over Chile had taken this exam, and he had emerged with the top score. Our family was justifiably thrilled, and I was as happy for him as if the triumph had been my own. He entered the engineering program at the university, and I started medical school. My problems began when, once the academic year had started, some of those in the medical school assumed that I was the young man with the highest score. They began to watch me (or at least I thought they did) to see if my academic performance met their expectations. Of course, I was not able to live up to the standards I assumed everyone had set for me, and as I was overly sensitive and of an obliging nature, for a long time I suffered low self-esteem. I sometimes just wanted to dig a hole and bury myself in it, but I did not give up. I think my persistence was due, in part, to the tenacity that is so characteristic of immigrant families like mine, which had come from Croatia (like so many in my country), but also to the lack of academic

---

12 In psychiatry, the terms *egosyntonic* and *egodystonic* are opposites. In layman's terms, they refer to what a person accepts or rejects as a part of him- or herself. *Egosyntonic* denotes a phenomenon that is accepted as natural to oneself and that is experienced as an appropriate response to a situation. *Egodystonic*, in contrast, alludes to a phenomenon that is rejected as something alien, imposed, against one's own nature.

alternatives for young people, regardless of social class, that was typical of Chile in those years. Until the 1990s, when private universities began to spring up around the country, it was almost inconceivable for a student to drop out of college, and changing majors was only a remote possibility. And so it was that tenacity became one of my closest friends during my first years at medical school, and if I have been able to achieve some of the goals I set for myself years ago, it is to a great extent thanks to the quality, so underestimated today, of perseverance.

Another incident from back then that comes to mind is the time when a classmate suggested that we study mathematics together. I suspect he assumed that I was a brilliant student and could teach him the material. He would not take no for an answer, so one day we settled down with our books for a study session at my house. However, I could not hide my own difficulty with the math problems, and it soon became clear that *I* was the one who needed help from *him*. Unfortunately, it was around that time, in 1974, that local university students became extremely competitive with one another, and abruptly so, it seems to me. This competitiveness was encouraged in part by the military junta that had recently taken power; fearing student protests against the coup, the new government increased academic demands to extreme levels, hoping to keep us at home with our books. In any case, my classmate walked out of my house as soon as he realized I would be of no help, unwittingly contributing to my inner discouragement. In the end, it was only through great effort and perseverance that I managed to pass my first year of medical school. My grades improved as time went by, but my success in those first years of college came at a high psychological cost as a consequence of both my poor high school preparation and my natural tendency to blush. If I had to sum up the cost, I would say that it was an unpleasant feeling of inadequacy that took me years to overcome.

Convinced as I am that those reading this book looking for help will identify with my experiences, I would like to add that all through my university years I tried numerous defense or camouflage techniques in an attempt to hide my propensity to blush. As soon as spring came and the days became sunnier, I would spend hours sunbathing to develop a tan that would hide the flushing, which not only ruined my day with alarming frequency but also caused me to live my life in a state of permanent anxiety.

I felt as if I were constantly walking a tightrope. A few months after graduation I grew a beard to hide my face, but it did little to disguise my blushing. In later chapters, when we look at other sufferers' testimonies, we will see other strategies for coping with PB. But here is perhaps one of the strangest techniques I tried in the early years of my struggle: Knowing that it was unexpected situations that were most likely to set my face aflame—someone suddenly appearing at my side to say hello, for example—I got into the habit of always being the one to initiate a greeting. That way no one would take me by surprise. In meetings or in large groups of people, I tended to stay in the background, but on the street or in hospital corridors I was always on the alert to be the first one to say hello to anyone who might be passing by. An unexpected side effect of this behavior was that it allowed me to make many friends and acquaintances so that, years later while walking one day through Salvador Hospital in Santiago with a former classmate, I was greeted by so many people that he suggested I run for public office! In my experiences with people who have sought help for excessive blushing, I have occasionally met patients who have used the same defense mechanism. I am unaware as to whether it is a conscious or an unconscious device.

For a decade now, I have been meeting with and attempting to treat many people suffering from the same problem that afflicted me for so many years and for which, until recently, no treatment was available. Today there are several possible treatments for both the more widely known social anxiety disorder (SAD), or social phobia, of which facial reddening is a symptom (see chapter 3), and for non-SAD-related PB. However, little is still known of these disorders, even among health professionals. This, in addition to the fact that these patients rarely consult their doctors, explains why most sufferers unfortunately go untreated.

Chapter 2
A Letter to My Doctor

Epistola enim non erubescit.
A letter doesn't blush.

—Cicero

I wrote the following letter at the end of June 2003:

Santiago, June 27, 2003
To: Dr. Claudio Suárez
Dear Claudio,

I am a colleague of yours, a specialist in psychiatry. I recently read the report on endoscopic[13] sympathectomy,[14] published in *El Mercurio*.[15] I felt identified in the article and hopeful after I finished it, probably like many other patients who have come to see you after reading the piece. While I had learned of the operation some time ago on the Internet, I was surprised to find out how simple the procedure is and have decided to consult with you. I

---

13 In this case, the term *endoscopic* refers to the fact that the operation involves a small incision to introduce a tube, or endoscope, into the body to view the chest cavity.

14 The word *sympathectomy* is derived from the Greek *sympathein* (to feel for) and *ektome* (excision). The term refers to the excision of a portion of the sympathetic nervous system, one of the two subdivisions of the autonomic nervous system. You will find further information on this surgical procedure in chapters 4 and 5.

15 The leading daily newspaper in Santiago, Chile.

am writing this letter simply because doing so helps me organize my ideas, and this way I can be sure I don't forget anything when we speak this afternoon.

All my life, but particularly since adolescence, I have suffered from profuse blushing and hand sweating at the slightest provocation. This has caused me a great deal of emotional distress, which I believe I have kept manageable through enormous willpower and the help of medication, which I will explain below. But I still have difficulty; thus my appointment with you this afternoon. From your work with other patients, you are undoubtedly aware of the psychological implications this problem has had in my life. I remember automatically blushing as a teenager when climbing aboard a city bus and feeling the other passengers' eyes on me, and more than once I let the bus go by when I felt that I might be the subject of scrutiny for some reason. My sweaty hands would leave damp marks on test papers when I was nervous; plastic folders, which do not absorb moisture, were particularly hazardous. Of course, the peace handshake during Mass[16] has also been a trial for me.

I felt extremely inhibited as a teenager by my blushing. Despite being reasonably good-looking and friendly, I rarely had a steady girlfriend because of my symptoms, which I found severely constraining. I turned almost instinctively at times to alcohol to calm my nerves, as do many people with this type of disorder, and while I fortunately never fell into depression, the hyperactivity of my autonomic nervous system has caused me a great deal of suffering. Extreme anxiety, particularly in social settings, has been a constant in my life, and even now, at my age, I suffer unnecessarily from this symptom.

---

16 The Catholic practice of the peace handshake involves shaking hands solemnly but fraternally with those sitting nearby during Mass. For palmar hyperhidrosis patients, this apparently simple gesture can be a torment.

At medical school I was always rather introverted (I didn't dare ask questions or otherwise participate in classes), but was well liked and accepted, or at least I felt that I was. My long hours of academic efforts paid off: I earned one of the highest scores in the country when I graduated, and I was granted the only psychiatry residency scholarship available that year. Up until that time, I had never taken anxiolytics or tranquilizers, but after three years of studying psychiatry in England,[17] I soon realized that life would be very difficult if I didn't get some help. I found myself required to take on some rather high-profile positions and responsibilities, and the mere thought of suffering visible and uncontrollable physical symptoms while in the public eye, and which I did frequently endure, brought on waves of anxiety. I sought help with a couple of psychiatrists, and my life changed when I discovered anxiolytics. Thanks in part to benzodiazepines and beta-blockers (which I take regularly when I have to teach a class, attend a directors' meeting,[18] or appear in a television interview), but primarily to willpower (telling myself, "This isn't going to get the better of me!"), I have been able to have a successful career, get married, and have two beautiful children.

You probably know that selective serotonin reuptake inhibitors (SSRIs), such as fluoxetine, paroxetine, and

---

17 I specialized in psychiatry in London at the Maudsley Hospital. Contrary to what one might think, I believe that my stay in the United Kingdom, far from helping me overcome my problem with blushing, actually exacerbated it. Cross-cultural research has shown that the rate of blushing reported by the English in embarrassing situations (55 percent) is the highest among all the countries studied. In England, embarrassment and blushing are important cultural constructs. It could almost be said that for the English, being looked at (especially if the gaze lasts longer than is considered appropriate) is almost akin to aggression. It is interesting to note that the British rate of averting one's gaze when embarrassed (41 percent) is much higher than that reported by Italians (8 percent) or Japanese (11 percent). See M. R. Leary et al. (1992).

18 I was secretary of the Neurology, Psychiatry, and Neurosurgery Society of Chile at the time I wrote the letter.

sertraline are used quite successfully to treat anxiety disorders. In my case and in those of some of my patients, while these medications do relieve anxiety, they have the very unpleasant side effect of causing sweating in the hands and feet (hand perspiration is a serious problem; foot sweating I don't mind).

In sum, I would like to evaluate with you the possibility of surgical treatment. I feel that the costs of continuing with this problem are high: suffering anxiety, having to take medication, and, despite my age, continuing to blush. I am tired of hearing comments (not ill-intentioned, but nonetheless irritating), such as "There you go up the cherry tree again, Doctor," and others you have undoubtedly heard before. In addition, in October I may be starting a two-year term as president of the Neurology, Psychiatry, and Neurosurgery Society, and I would like to minimize the likelihood that these problems will continue.

I have, of course, read about the surgical procedure; this is one of the main topics I would like to discuss with you. I do not suffer from axillary hyperhidrosis, and I find hyperhidrosis of the feet tolerable.[19] I have heard that the surgery has best results with palmar hyperhidrosis and facial reddening, which are precisely the two difficulties with which I struggle the most.

Finally, I appreciate your opinion and guidance in this matter.

Enrique Jadresic

P.S. I would prefer that you return this letter to me after reading it.[20]

---

19 Hyperhidrosis is a primary illness; that is, it is of spontaneous origin rather than secondary to another disorder. It causes excessive sweating, generally on the hands, face, feet, and armpits under normal physiological conditions.

20 As I maybe should have expected, I forgot to ask Claudio Suárez for the letter once he had read it, probably due to the anxiety I was feeling when I met with him that first day. I assume it had remained among my medical records. Dr. Suárez later had the letter discreetly returned to me.

Chapter 3
Is Pathological Blushing an Illness?

All human beings blush at some time. It is a universal experience, one that is characteristic of the human race. Charles Darwin, the English naturalist, in his 1872 book *The Expression of the Emotions in Man and Animals*, held that blushing is "the most peculiar and the most human of all expressions."[21] He devotes an entire chapter to the topic of blushing, a phenomenon, as he says, that consists of a reddening of the face (especially the cheeks), ears, and neck, and occasionally other parts of the body, brought on by the "thinking of what others think of us." In a more recent review, the blush experience is defined as "a spontaneous reddening or darkening of the face, ears, neck, and upper chest that occurs in response to perceived social scrutiny or evaluation."[22] The term *flushing* refers to the same phenomenon, but without the psychological component.[23] Both blushing and flushing can be accompanied by a sensation of heat in the affected area.

Nowadays, in an age when criticisms or questions have arisen in various fields as to the "medicalization"[24] of life, it seems to me not only legitimate

---

21 See C. Darwin (1872/1955).

22 See M. R. Leary et al. (1992).

23 See D. Ray and G. Williams (1993).

24 *Medicalization* refers to the process through which nonmedical problems are defined and treated as medical issues. Some people have questioned the pertinence of incorporating into the medical field such problems as menopause, aging, some sexual dysfunctions, jet lag, caffeine intoxication, and alcoholism. For further discussion on the topic, see P. Conrad (2007).

but also appropriate, to pose a few questions: Can blushing really be considered an illness? Mightn't it be just an invention of professionals who benefit from selling pharmacological treatments and other options, even surgery? Isn't it another manifestation of the "medicalization" of human behavior? These are certainly valid questions delving into deep, complex issues, even philosophical ones. While the purpose of this book is not to answer these questions in full, I would like to make a few observations.

My viewpoint is that all human illnesses, whether diabetes or schizophrenia, are man-made creations. There are no real illnesses, only operational concepts that we use to describe natural phenomena because they are useful in alleviating human suffering and in communicating with others. In other words, we can say that when certain natural phenomena affect us negatively, we call them illnesses. This is true for all pathologies, whether we are dealing, for example, with viral diseases or psychiatric disorders, such as depression. Thus, the presence of the flu virus in an individual's organism does not constitute an illness; it is only when the person begins to show symptoms that we can talk of disease. Likewise, feeling sad is not the same as being depressed, unless the sadness is very intense and/or occurs with other symptoms and prevents the person from leading a normal life. When this occurs, we call it "clinical depression" and treat it as we would pain or a fever. Facial reddening induced by psychological stimuli is a similar situation. The simple act of blushing cannot be called an illness or disorder. Moreover, turning red in certain situations is not only appropriate but expected. This is normal blushing. In my opinion, facial reddening can be considered a morbid symptom or a psychiatric disorder only when it is brought on by minor psychological precipitants, causes psychological suffering, and interferes significantly with a person's academic/occupational functioning or interpersonal relationships. In these cases, it can be treated if the patient so desires.

Curiously, the scientific literature does not normally differentiate between the two types of blushing described above, between normal blushing that is expected in certain contexts and does not limit the individual and blushing that causes emotional pain and interferes with the person's daily life, thus constituting an abnormality or disorder. For the latter, I coined the term *pathological blushing* (PB) for the first edition of this book since, until that time, the conceptual distinction between normal facial blushing and its pathological counterpart had not yet been described. I hope that the cases presented in the second part of this book will convince readers of the need to distinguish conceptually between the two types of facial reddening.[25]

A second consideration is whether PB is a symptom or a sign. In medicine, the term *symptom* refers to a patient's subjective reference to a perception or change that he or she can recognize as anomalous or caused by a pathological state or disease. A *sign*, in contrast, is the objective (nonsubjective) evidence of a disease or disorder. I believe that, when considering PB from a clinical point of view, both aspects, subjective experience and objective evidence, should be included. In this respect, Edelmann has posited that individuals with chronic facial blushing (what we would call PB) may be differentiated from normal blushers in four ways:[26]

First, they may be more susceptible physiologically, with variables, such as heart rate and body temperature more sensitive to physical activity or stress. Second, they may blush more visibly; some studies (not all) show that these individuals turn a brighter red than non-PB patients. Third, they may by nature be more inclined to focus on their thoughts and bodily reactions. Last, and possibly linked to the third, they may tend to be overly concerned about both the blushing itself and the possibility of it.

In other words, Edelmann says, while chronic blushers may redden more easily and more visibly, this characteristic is not necessarily at the root of what causes the embarrassment. One crucial factor seems to be the fact that those who blush chronically are frequently more sensitive to their body's reactions, pay more attention to them, and have a greater fear of blushing. In this sense, it is interesting to reiterate that while embarrassment usually accompanies blushing, the two do not necessarily

---

25 Leary et al. have described two types of facial reddening from another point of view: first, the typical blush, which appears quickly (in a matter of seconds) on the face, neck, and ears, and spreads uniformly over the affected areas; and second, the "creeping blush," which occurs more slowly, appearing first as red splotches, usually on the upper chest or lower neck. As the minutes go by, it spreads upward onto the upper neck, jaws, and cheeks. Even at its peak, a creeping blush is blotchy rather than uniform in color. See M. R. Leary et al. (1992) or Alfredo H. Cía (2004).
26 See R. J. Edelmann (1990/2004)

go hand in hand. In fact, although they are atypical, there are people who blush without feeling the anxiety of chronic blushers; contrariwise, there are people who can feel embarrassment without turning red.

From the psychiatric perspective, Pierre Janet (1903), in a pioneering work on phobias, identified variations of what he called *social phobias*, including *erythrophobia* (fear of blushing). However, within today's concepts of mental disorders, the illness most associated with facial blushing is social anxiety disorder (SAD), formerly known as social phobia (I will use both terms interchangeably here). This disorder affects 13 percent of the population at some time in their lives. According to one study, up to 50 percent of SAD patients say they blush frequently.[27] But even individuals with social phobia who do not blush experience the same phenomena that go along with facial reddening: feeling embarrassed, averting the gaze, withdrawing attention from the observer or speaker, and, in many cases, smiling or grinning nervously.

The tenth version of the World Health Organization's International Statistical Classification of Diseases and Related Health Problems (ICD-10)[28] defines social phobia, or SAD, as a marked fear of being the center of attention or of behaving in an embarrassing or humiliating way, leading to social avoidance. The American Psychiatric Association's Diagnostic and Statistical Manual (DSM-5)[29] characterizes SAD as the presence of persistent, marked anxiety in different social or public situations for fear that they might be embarrassing. So, then, if blushing and its emotional concomitants are a normal component of SAD, why does this book focus on facial reddening, and specifically on that with a pathological connotation (PB), rather than on SAD? There are various reasons.

The main reason is that while I have written this book as a physician, the purpose of the text is to discuss the concerns of patients, and patients are distressed, not by SAD per se, but by the telltale color in their cheeks. Similarly, a mother caring for her children, or anyone whose health suddenly deteriorates, is primarily concerned, at least at first, with the listlessness, fever, pain, or anxiety and how to cure it rather than by the

---

27 See P. L. Amies et al. (1983).

28 See World Health Organization (1993).

29 See American Psychiatric Association (2013).

theory and knowledge structure that doctors have built around a specific ailment. In other words, the individual was not made for the medical world, but quite the reverse.

A second reason for focusing specifically on blushing is to draw attention to a phenomenon that is generally trivialized and nearly always assumed to be a normal experience when, in fact, that experience can actually become a symptom (a situation that can be determined only through careful evaluation). When this is the case, options for treatment should be explored if the patient so desires, which is usually the reason a person seeks medical help.

Third, the general belief that today's psychiatric diagnostic criteria correspond to actually existing biological conditions is an illusion. The Spanish psychiatrist Julio Sanjuan has probed this question based on the enormous paradox that we do not yet have a single biological marker that is specific enough to be included within the diagnostic criteria of even one psychiatric disorder. This is why many researchers today look more into the correlation of concrete symptoms, such as hallucinations, lack of concentration, and anxiety rather than the biology behind the illnesses of uncertain nosology included in today's classifications.[30] Thus it would be perfectly reasonable to look for the biological factor(s) correlative to PB.

Finally, while our experience has shown that PB commonly occurs with SAD, chronic blushers can suffer certain symptoms of social anxiety without fulfilling all the criteria required for that diagnosis.

Evolutionary Perspective

It is enlightening to note that although Darwin recognized he could not explain the phenomenon of facial reddening, the evolutionary (or evolutionist) viewpoint of psychology or psychiatry has established correlations between human blushing and the appeasement displays exhibited by certain animals. In effect, the animals' display behaviors reduce the possibility of an attack by members of their own species. Likewise, human blushing is considered to reduce negative reactions on the

---

30 See J. Sanjuan (2000).

part of observers.[31] In the past, and even now in some cultures, blushing is associated with modesty and charm. Neither can we overlook how many women use cosmetics to simulate blushing cheeks, a custom that has persisted in numerous cultures over the centuries.

In view of this evolutionary logic, one might ask why, if blushing serves to defuse a threat, people so want to avoid it. For the few doctors who work in this area, our experience has shown us that most patients seek help not because of normal, occasional facial reddening, which we know is a natural part of life, but because they blush excessively and at socially inappropriate times. They turn bright red when they least expect it: when running into an acquaintance on the street, talking on the telephone, or even in front of family members. Blushing is better tolerated when it seems socially appropriate, such as when people receive public recognition or have "Happy Birthday" sung to them. It is turning red for no apparent reason that causes such distress. Blushers may fear that others believe they are hiding a misdeed (e.g., blushing when they are teased about something they have ostensibly done in private), or they may worry about seeming to lose their composure in nonthreatening situations, thus being considered shy, awkward, or, in today's jargon, a loser.

The evolutionary perspective suggests that pathological anxiety has arisen from humankind's naturally evolved disposition to monitor and react to threats, which in some people has become, in a sense, an off-balance "fight or flight" mechanism that errs by overprotecting against perceived threats. A similar alteration may underlie pathological blushing. In other words, in some people the evolutionary defense mechanism has become an "overreactive" emotional response or a system that erroneously causes, as a result of minor stimuli, the facial coloration we see in our patients, as well as the cognitive distortions and irrational thoughts that so frequently accompany it.

From a different, but also evolutionary, focus, it has been suggested that there are actually many more than a dozen or so emotions (normally there are considered to be between seven and twelve). These would include the self-conscious emotions of embarrassment, shame, and guilt, all of

---

31 See D. J. Stein and C. Bouwer (1997).

which facilitate adherence to social norms,[32] as well as other emotions, such as compassion or gratitude, that are crucial to successful interpersonal relations.

Finally, I have been pleased to see that medical journals have begun to publish more articles on blushing, sometimes taking the symptom outside of the SAD context.[33] This development does not invalidate, as I have said, the fact that PB usually appears as just one component, albeit a primary one, of SAD. I see the medical community's increasing concern for facial reddening, particularly when it is debilitating and interferes with a normal life, as a positive step. This new concern has served, for example, to create awareness that there are also nonemotional causes of what is sometimes called "blushing," although the term "flushing" should actually be used to denote facial coloration that occurs without a psychological basis. I mention this distinction because these possibilities should always be ruled out when a patient seeks medical help. For example, we know that exercise or ambient heat can cause physiological facial vasodilation, and that episodes of postmenopausal facial redness, which are called hot flashes and are associated with lowered levels of estrogen, have no psychological connotation. In addition, many medications, and even alcohol, can bring on reddening, as can some foods. Sometimes rosacea, a dermatological problem, can be preceded by a prolonged tendency to blush.[34] Finally, rare systemic diseases, such as carcinoid syndrome and mastocytosis, can trigger flushing but, again, without the underlying emotional causes.

---

32 Greater adherence to social norms facilitates social cohesion. The other side of the coin would be individuals who are less susceptible to self-conscious emotions and who, it is suggested, are more prone to antisocial behaviors. Authors such as C. Darwin and E. Goffman put forth variations of this hypothesis many years ago. Not for nothing are people who fail to meet social standards called "shameless."

33 See M. Nicolau (2006).

34 Rosacea, or acne rosacea, is a chronic inflammatory skin disorder of the cheeks, nose, chin, forehead, or eyelids. It may cause a reddened appearance, spider veins, inflammation, or acne-like blemishes. Rosacea occurs more frequently among fair-skinned people who blush easily, usually women, although men tend to have more severe cases. There is no cure, but it can generally be controlled through proper treatment. In my clinical practice with blushing patients, I have seen numerous individuals who have been treated by dermatologists.

Chapter 4
Returning to Clinical Practice

Psychiatry is the most scientific of the humanities and the
most humanistic of the sciences.

—Sir Martin Roth

My life seemed to go into fast-forward after I visited Dr. Suárez and gave
him the letter I had written that morning. My intuition was correct: after
the usual medical evaluation, the doctor confirmed that I was a good
candidate for surgery and that the operation would probably help me. A
month later, at the end of July 2003 and with all the necessary tests in
hand, I underwent surgery. I told no one but my wife; so embarrassing is
the whole issue of facial blushing that I never even considered discussing
it with anyone else. Only after four years did I finally tell my mother
about the operation when the subject of my lifelong struggle with blushing
came up during an evening conversation. I sent her an e-mail at the time,
dodging the issue, saying, "Could it be that as we get older it's easier to
talk about things that we used to keep to ourselves?" In reality, while I
do believe that it is easier to talk about our feelings and acknowledge
our fears later in life, my delay in telling her about the surgery came
down to a very simple explanation: I was embarrassed to tell her I had
had surgery for blushing. On the other hand, I was not embarrassed, or
much less so, to reveal that palmar hyperhidrosis was the other reason for
the operation. In our world today, with its unrestrained competitiveness,
extreme reductionisms, and simplistic distinctions between "winners" and

"losers," it is difficult for us to confess our feelings of inadequacy, even to those who love us unconditionally.

Now let's stop and consider something for a moment. What the suffering *means* to the patient as an individual is crucial in this context, and it is an aspect of the human experience that the medical world all too frequently overlooks, especially when dealing with a disorder about which little is known. We frequently forget that the doctor's and patient's priorities do not necessarily coincide. In my work with PB patients, I have repeatedly noticed that in their previous encounters with health-care professionals, physician and patient did not necessarily seem to "be on the same page." Interviews with patients have given me the impression that in previous consultations with doctors, the patient felt overwhelmed, seemingly engulfed by the affliction. At the same time, I am sure the health professional was perplexed, his or her difficulty stemming not so much from the need to incorporate new ideas as from the need to let go of the old ones, especially in making a diagnosis. Clearly, it is essential to identify and classify the illness, but anyone who, like the psychiatrist, works primarily through interpersonal encounters has the unavoidable obligation to discover the deeper meaning that the patient places on the ailment (and even on life itself) while making a diagnosis.

Returning to my own case, I would like to stress the fact that even while I knew, rationally, that I could count on the unconditional support of those close to me, at first I found it impossible to share with them events in my life of which they were completely unaware. In fact, my father and brothers learned of my surgery only when they read the first edition of this book. Many readers may find it an easy matter to confide in their loved ones and reach out for help, but for those who feel more intensely (or are overly concerned with) the self-conscious emotions, such as embarrassment, shame, or guilt, it is extraordinarily difficult to put the experience into words. And loneliness is just one short step away. As someone once said, just as illness is the greatest of miseries, loneliness is the worst consequence of illness.[35]

As my own case evolved, after years of suffering from something I

---

35 The statement belongs to John Donne, who was quoted by Oliver Sacks in his book *Awakenings*, page 22. See O. Sacks (1987).

could not control and had not dared to share with anyone, I suddenly discovered that many others were immersed in the same miserable, endless silence, a muteness most do not have the courage to break, because of unjustified fear. Even though they have done nothing wrong, they are afraid of being misunderstood.

I had a few minor complications after the sympathectomy, mainly a certain irritation in the trachea and a slight hypersensitivity in the chest and back. Unfortunately, as the days went by, I also developed intercostal neuritis,[36] which, besides causing an intense, constant burning pain for several weeks, worried me greatly because I knew as a doctor that sometimes this sort of pain does not subside. I vividly remember that the slightest touch of clothing on my skin increased the pain to indescribable agony. I used a woman's nipple guard to fashion a transparent shield that I taped to my right areola to prevent the slightest touch of my shirt on the nipple; I wore this for several days. I try not to exaggerate, and I certainly do not want to sound like a raving psychiatrist, but I felt as if a burning lance were stabbing into the right side of my torso through the nipple.[37] I reflected on the experience of pain many times during those weeks, and I began to understand how people come to commit suicide because of intolerable physical pain. Fortunately, the pain disappeared after a few weeks. Was the relief due in part to the numerous medications my doctor prescribed (high doses of powerful painkillers like carbamazepine or gabapentin)? I do not know and, looking at it from my viewpoint as patient, I have to admit that I do not care.

Just forty-eight hours after the surgery, I returned to my usual, albeit sporadic, teaching at the Graduate School of Medicine at the University of Chile in Santiago. I do not remember the first class I taught after the operation, but looking back, I assume I took a tranquilizer, as I had done for years, to calm the anxiety I still felt when standing in front of a class,

---

36 Intercostal neuritis is an inflammation of an intercostal nerve. It causes pain, frequently intense, in the torso or arm, or in the skin of these areas. It has several causes, including the sympathectomy. It is not a common complication of the surgery, but when it does occur after the operation, it usually disappears within three to six weeks.

37 I should point out that, due to a previous lesion in my right lung, the surgeon opted for entering the torso through the right nipple rather than through the armpit, which is the usual procedure.

despite my years of teaching. Even though the benefits of the surgery were soon apparent, I discovered that it takes time to become accustomed to a lower level of vigilance and alarm after three decades of living in a state of heightened nervous expectation.

I clearly remember my ambivalence when Dr. Suárez asked me to evaluate a PB and palmar hyperhidrosis patient just one week after my operation. I was flattered at his request and happy at the idea of helping someone suffering from the same problem I was. But at the same time, I was not sure if I was up to the challenge of plunging once more into a situation dealing with the same ailment from which I was trying so hard to escape. Still, I told my colleague that he could count on me. I had not planned to work with him on a regular basis, but I immediately acceded to his request out of a deep sense of gratitude. Despite my mixed feelings, I soon realized I had made the right decision.

Just before the appointment with that first patient, I found myself, after nearly twenty years of psychiatric experience, with a case of nerves, almost as if it were my first day in medical practice. I had undergone the surgery, and supposedly I had acquired a certain immunity (even though I knew that after the operation the blushing becomes more sporadic and lessens in intensity rather than disappearing completely). Still, there was no denying it: I was nervous. Despite the operation, my greatest fear still was blushing. But that day, it did not happen.

Even so, my insecurity lingered through the next few evaluations I did for Dr. Suárez. One underlying factor, I believe, was my indecision as to whether to share my own experience with the patients. After all, the only people who knew about my problem were the surgical team and my wife; even the rest of my family remained unaware.

Fortunately, I soon became less sensitive to the stimuli that had previously brought on the episodes of blushing. My confidence soared, and almost before I knew it, I began to tell my patients that I had undergone surgery. Besides, I seemed to know intuitively what to do as I began to deal with more blushing cases. I very soon gave Dr. Suárez permission to tell his patients that the psychiatrist who was going to evaluate them had suffered through the same difficulties and had also been his patient on the operating table. I became happy to share my secret with the patients; it was gratifying to know that they felt understood and to hear them say so. Many of them had visited numerous specialists—dermatologists, neurologists, psychiatrists, psychologists, hypnotists, and more—but rarely had they felt that the health-care professional understood their condition. The doctors had sincerely tried to help, but without success. I also discovered that on the few occasions when the patients brought up the possibility of surgery, the doctors usually minimized the importance of the symptom, and they categorically and immediately ruled out the option of surgery.

Since then, I have, as a physician and psychiatrist, evaluated many PB patients who have gone to Dr. Suárez for surgery, and I have become convinced that a psychiatric evaluation is necessary. I have tried to accompany the patients whenever possible, if not in person, then by e-mail, through the process that many of them refer to as "taking their foot off the brake." It is almost as if they had been wearing an invisible straitjacket for years that restrained them from living a full life, from embracing the world. I am grateful to the noble profession that I chose, which, in a twist of fate, has led me in recent years to work with and help fellow sufferers.

I have stayed in contact with many of these patients over time, generally through e-mail. I have heard the personal stories of hundreds of people, all of them meaningful. Many of them are powerful and encouraging, but a few are full of unmitigated pain and frustration. After the success of the first edition of this book, I learned of many more. Deep down, I now feel that I have done something important: I have been able to help validate the suffering of those misunderstood men and women who, with reason or otherwise, struggle to free themselves from the fire in their cheeks.

Chapter 5

Options for Treating Social Anxiety Disorder/Social Phobia and Pathological Blushing

It is important to remember that simply feeling anxiety in social situations does not warrant medical treatment. Currently, social phobia is diagnosed only when social situations are avoided or endured with intense fear or anxiety.

Although the benefits of early treatment for social anxiety disorder (SAD) are clear, many patients do not seek help until they have developed complications, such as severe depression or substance abuse, usually involving alcohol. SAD patients rarely seek help for blushing; when they do, it is usually after finding information on the Internet.

Research supports the use of two treatments for social phobia: certain medications and a specific method of psychotherapy called cognitive behavioral therapy (CBT), which consists primarily of gradual exposure to the feared situation.

Drug Therapy for SAD/Social Phobia

For cases of SAD, many experts consider selective serotonin reuptake inhibitors (SSRIs), a type of medication whose effects include increasing levels of the neurotransmitter serotonin, to be the pharmacological treatment of choice. These drugs include paroxetine, sertraline, fluoxetine, citalopram, escitalopram, and fluvoxamine. A recent study among SAD patients with erythrophobia showed that treatment with citalopram decreased their phobia symptoms by 60 percent.[38] Although these medications are generally well tolerated, they do have side effects, especially during the first weeks of treatment, when they can temporarily cause headaches, nausea, and insomnia. In addition, they frequently reduce sexual desire and delay orgasm, symptoms that only sometimes decrease or disappear over time.

Another type of medication, selective noradrenalin and serotonin reuptake inhibitors (SNSRIs), such as venlafaxine and duloxetine, have also proved to be effective. Of course, these medications can cause side effects as well. The results of studies with other compounds, such as gabapentin and pregabalin have also been encouraging.[39]

For cases in which symptoms of SAD occur only when one has to speak or otherwise perform in public, drugs, such as beta-blockers (propranolol, atenolol) or benzodiazepines (alprazolam, lorazepam) that are taken occasionally and only as needed have traditionally been considered effective.

Another recent study among women shows that a neurosteroid administered as a nasal spray and taken only as needed is also helpful in situations of acute social anxiety. This preliminary finding is very promising since, if it is confirmed, it would show that minute doses (called nanomolars) of a medication can be used since they act directly through nasal receptors rather than going through the circulatory system.[40]

Psychotherapy for SAD/Social Phobia

Scientific evidence shows that cognitive behavioral therapy (CBT), a form of psychotherapy used to treat several anxiety disorders, is especially effective in treating panic disorder and SAD. It consists of two components, one cognitive and the other behavioral. The *cognitive component* helps people become aware of their thought patterns and then make the changes needed to overcome their fears. For example, social phobia patients can learn to

---

38 See A. Pelissolo and A. Moukheiber (2013).

39 See A. C. Pande et al. (2004).

40 See M. R. Liebowitz et al. (2014).

question the belief that they are constantly being observed and judged by others. The *behavioral component* seeks to change patients' reactions to the situations that cause anxiety. A key element of this component is gradual exposure, with individuals confronting the situations they fear in a careful, structured manner. The purpose is also to have the patients learn new behaviors by teaching them to respond to the situations in a different way and then monitor their reactions. The treatment is implemented with the guidance and support of the therapist once he or she and the patient are both confident that the conditions are right. CBT for social phobia also involves anxiety management training, which may include breathing techniques and relaxation exercises that can be practiced *in situ*. The therapy can take place partially in a group context, allowing the patients to share their experiences. Group therapy also helps them develop a feeling of being accepted by others and gives them an opportunity to confront their behavioral challenges in a nonthreatening situation. Some studies suggest that social skills training can be useful in treating SAD. It is not clear, however, whether specific techniques and practices are needed, or if the individual simply needs support with social functioning in general and in dealing with anxiety-ridden social situations.

Drug Therapy for PB

A study by Connor et al.[41] is especially interesting for the issue of blushing, one of the reasons that SAD patients seek medical help. This was the first scientifically rigorous study (double-blind and placebo-controlled, in scientific terminology) to demonstrate the effectiveness of a drug, specifically sertraline, in treating social anxiety–related blushing.

My colleagues and I conducted our own study of patients with SAD who sought help for blushing. We compared the results on intense facial blushing among patients who took sertraline with those among patients who underwent surgery and others who did not receive any treatment. The patients reported that both the medication and the surgery, although the latter to a greater extent, are efficacious in treating facial blushing.[42]

---

41 See K. M. Connor et al. (2006).
42 See E. Jadresic et al. (2011).

Other drugs that have been used to treat blushing are beta-blockers, which help control the physical symptoms of anxiety and, more specifically, because studies have shown that the acute stage of blushing is regulated primarily by beta-adrenergic sympathetic nerves, which are responsible for the dilation of blood vessels in the face.[43,44] These medications can be used on an ongoing basis (atenolol, metoprolol, propranolol) or only occasionally (propranolol). In our experience, 20 to 40 milligrams of propranolol, taken along with 0.25 milligram of alprazolam forty to sixty minutes prior to a situation that typically triggers blushing, is usually quite effective. Our patients often call this the "magic combination." It is a good treatment option, but it has the drawback that if patients are able to deal successfully with social situations, they tend to attribute the success to the medication rather than taking the credit themselves. In other words, it is a strategy that reinforces the use of drugs rather than cognitive behavioral techniques, which, as we will soon see, involve learning processes.

Clonidine, an adrenergic agonist typically used to treat high blood pressure, has been found over time to have other uses, such as alleviating menopausal hot flashes. It has also been used to treat facial blushing.[45]

Finally, a recent study suggests, interestingly, that ibuprofen, a widely used anti-inflammatory, reduces blushing (arising in situations of discomfiture or embarrassment) when applied to the cheeks in gel form. It also seems to help control flushing caused by exertion. Ibuprofen works by decreasing the formation of prostaglandins, substances that contribute to the inflammatory processes in the face that result in blushing.[46]

Psychotherapy for PB

Using psychotherapy to help patients control their blushing in social situations can be complex, and it is important to find a therapist who has been trained to apply the specific methods that have been proved to be effective. In general, the same techniques are used as for treating SAD, or social phobia. These techniques, rather than trying to decrease the intensity

43 See S. Mellander et al. (1982).
44 See P. D. Drummond and J. W. Lance (1987).
45 See C. van der Meer (1985).
46 See P. D. Drummond et al. (2013).

and/or frequency of the episodes of facial blushing, focus on controlling the fear of blushing, or erythrophobia. This process indirectly helps people to blush less, as the expectation of blushing has been proved to act as a self-fulfilling prophecy and can actually lead to facial reddening.[47]

Task Concentration Training (TCT)

Until now, there have been only two or three therapeutic methods designed specifically to treat the fear of blushing. The most widely known is *task concentration training*, or TCT, developed by Bögels and her colleagues.[48] This technique is based on the idea that people who blush are too self-conscious during social interactions (excessively focused on their emotions, behavior, physical appearance, and level of activation) and pay little attention to the tasks at hand, the other(s) involved, and their surroundings. In these individuals, any sign of activity in their sympathetic nervous system, such as a faster heartbeat, perspiring hands, and—especially—warm cheeks, increases their focus on themselves. As their blushing becomes clearly visible to others, they become even more self-conscious.

Task concentration training therapy consists of teaching patients to direct their attention away from themselves when they blush and to focus on the tasks involved in the specific social interaction (waiting on customers, for example) rather than on themselves. The therapy consists of three stages: (1) becoming familiar with the processes of paying attention and becoming aware of the negative effects of increasing one's attention on oneself; (2) focusing one's attention away from oneself in nonthreatening situations (such as watching TV, making a phone call, walking in the park, or listening to the lyrics of a song); and (3) focusing one's attention away from oneself in threatening situations.

In the first stage, the patient learns how blushing and attention on oneself reinforce each other and how this interaction begins to produce anxiety, negative thoughts about oneself, problems concentrating, and awkwardness. Next, patients are shown how, by focusing their attention out (toward the tasks involved in the social action and their surroundings)

---

47 See P. D. Drummond (2001).
48 See S. M. Bögels et al. (1997).

rather than in, they can begin to break the vicious circle that perpetuates their blushing. Patients are asked to keep a daily record of their blushing episodes, noting how anxious they were and estimating what percentage of concentration was on themselves, on the interaction, and on their surroundings at that time. Patients do concentration exercises under the guidance of the therapist that involve both listening and telling stories. Later, these daily records are used in "homework" assigned by the therapist.

During the nonthreatening focusing exercises, patients are told, for example, to walk through a (quiet) park paying attention to all the stimuli around (visual, auditory, olfactory, kinesthetic) and in their own body. Patients are instructed to focus first on one aspect at a time, and then on all stimuli simultaneously (integrated attention). One homework assignment frequently given is to have a telephone conversation and then to summarize it.

To practice threatening situations, patients make a list of around ten social situations that are important in their life and that trigger blushing. The list is organized in an increasing hierarchy, in which the first item is the least threatening for the patient. The goal is for patients to concentrate on the task involved in each situation and to return their focus to the task every time they get distracted by (thinking of) blushing or by focusing on themselves. Whenever possible, these more complex exercises are practiced first in the therapist's office, but they later become homework assignments of which patients keep written records. Any difficulties that arise are discussed with the therapist in the following session.

Learning to concentrate on the task at hand is considered a coping strategy, and it must be taught by a properly trained therapist. The training is generally done in six to eight weekly sessions lasting forty-five to sixty minutes each.

Cognitive Behavioral Therapy

Once task concentration training has been completed, generally another six to eight weekly sessions are given on cognitive behavioral therapy (CBT). The procedure is similar to that used with patients suffering from SAD/social phobia, but special attention is paid to the safety-seeking behaviors that people adopt when they fear blushing but that are generally counterproductive. The therapy seeks to change these behaviors, which are generally things the person does, or does not do, in order to remain calm or to keep the blushing down, or at least less visible. One of the most common, of course, is avoiding or minimizing social contact, perhaps, for example, by sitting in the last row in a conference thinking that one might need to get up to go to the restroom. Other strategies are to use makeup, cover the face with hair, stand against the light, wear sunglasses, or grow a beard (for men). Others are more complex, such as trying to control every aspect of a presentation one is going to make: learning it by memory, making sure that the room is as dark as possible, taking a tranquilizer beforehand, etc.

I remember one patient who, every time she had to give a presentation in public, would spend the previous day in the sun without sunblock. This way, she argued, she *arrived* at the presentation red and thus avoided *turning* red. This behavior certainly entailed a risk to her health, but, in addition, it was not foolproof: naturally, the day prior to her presentation might be cloudy.

While these safety-seeking behaviors may provide some short-term relief for people who blush, in the end they are counterproductive because, if the catastrophes that the patients anticipate do not occur, they attribute it to these behaviors instead of concluding that the situation was less threatening than they had thought. In other words, these behaviors keep them from learning that the consequences they fear are actually distorted ideas, and it prevents them from adopting coping strategies that are more productive. Several techniques are used to reduce these behaviors, such as practicing with simulations or re-creations of each problematic situation before trying the skills learned in real-life circumstances.

Other therapies used with people who fear blushing are social skills training,[49] mindfulness-based cognitive therapy,[50] and paradoxical intention. This last technique consists of asking patients to blush when they feel that they are turning red, and it has also proved effective in decreasing the frequency of blushing in people with a chronic tendency to redden.[51]

---

49 See S. M. Bögels and M. Voncken (2008).
50 See J. Piet et al. (2010).
51 See J. A. Boeringa (1983).

Length of Treatment

Many people will wonder how long the treatment should last. For drug therapy, there is no scientifically based answer since, due to the high costs involved, studies generally cover only the first six months of medication use. Clinical practice, however, tends to show that people who stop taking the medication after that time are more likely to have the symptoms recur than do those who continue with the drug for longer periods of time. In my medical practice, I generally advise patients to continue with the treatment for about one to two years. I then gradually cut back on the medication and watch to see if symptoms reappear. If they do, I have the patient return to the original dosage for a more prolonged, or even indefinite, period of time.

Cognitive behavioral therapy (CBT), as we have seen, is a short-term treatment usually lasting only a few months. As it involves learning processes, it has the advantage of providing longer-lasting results.

One option to consider, since patients tend to respond more quickly to medication than to CBT, is to begin treatment using both methods simultaneously and, after a time, to gradually decrease the use of drugs. Another alternative is to begin with a course of drug therapy, cut back gradually after a time, and then immediately begin CBT to prevent symptoms from recurring.

Surgical Treatment for PB Associated with SAD/Social Phobia

For patients with severe, objectionable blushing that have not responded to CBT or drug therapy, another option to consider is *endoscopic thoracic sympathectomy*[52] (ETS), also known as *videothoracoscopic sympathectomy* (VTS). For the rest of the book, I will use only the former term. Briefly, the surgery is based on the discovery that these patients' sympathetic nervous systems do not work properly. For example, one research study associates erythrophobia with a tendency for the facial redness to dissipate more slowly.[53] My personal experience bears this out, since I realized soon after the operation that although I still blushed, albeit less intensely, the color

---

52 See NICE clinical guidelines (2014).
53 See P. D. Drummond et al. (2007).

was much more fleeting. This result relieved my anxiety, which, in turn, meant that I tended to blush more sporadically. This result is consistent with the explanation that ETS acts on a postcapillary sphincter to prevent the blood vessels in the face from retaining blood.[54]

Doctors learned of the benefits of the sympathectomy in treating facial sweating in the 1930s, and it has been known as a treatment for hand sweating since the fifties. The operation was proposed for treating facial blushing for the first time in 1985.[55] However, since it involved major surgery on both sides of the thorax (where the fibers of the sympathetic nervous system are located) the operation was almost impracticable. It was only in the 1990s, with the advent of videosurgery techniques (minimally invasive surgery and the use of special video cameras), that it became a simple procedure. ETS has become known to the Latin American medical field as a treatment for pathological blushing only in the last ten years.

The procedure is performed under general anesthesia in an operating room. An incision less than one inch long is made in the right armpit. A tiny video camera is then inserted, providing the surgeons with a clear view of the entire inside of the thorax.

A special instrument inserted through another small incision in the armpit is used to locate the chain of sympathetic ganglia; a small section of the sympathetic trunk is then severed and cauterized at the level of the second, third, or fourth rib. The T2 ganglion is severed for blushing and hyperhidrosis of the face. If hyperhidrosis of the hands is also a problem, T3 is cut as well. (If the patient suffers only from palmar hyperhidrosis, only T3 is cut.) If excessive sweating is also present in the armpits, the procedure is extended to include T4. (If the patient's only symptom is axillary hyperhidrosis, only T4 is severed.) A slender drainage tube is left for about two hours at the location of the first incision. The procedure is then repeated on the other side.

Although any surgery involves risks, the procedure is quite safe. The operation takes about an hour, and the patient generally remains hospitalized overnight. Some cases may be handled on an outpatient basis.

The symptoms improve rapidly, with the results of the operation

---

54 As explained to me by Dr. Claudio Suárez.
55 See R. Wittmoser (1985).

normally being seen within hours, days, or weeks. Most patients (80 to 90 percent) report a significant reduction in blushing and a definite improvement in their quality of life,[56] with decreased intensity, frequency, and/or duration of blushing episodes. For most individuals, this result translates into improved self-confidence, greater participation in social activities (which they used to avoid), and, not infrequently, improvements in their jobs and personal relationships.

The longest follow-up study done so far on patients who have undergone ETS covered 536 surgeries and showed a patient satisfaction rate of 73 percent after fourteen years. The study also showed that only quickly spreading blushing triggered by social situations responded well to the surgery. The authors believe that the decreased satisfaction among patients compared to that expressed after a shorter follow-up period may be due to the fact that their memories of blushing tend to fade over time, while the compensatory sweating persists.[57]

Complications are rare, but they have been reported.[58] The most frequent postoperative side effect (44 to 99 percent of patients)[59] is compensatory sweating, which is the tendency, usually permanent, to perspire more heavily in other parts of the body. It occurs mainly on the torso and, of course, intensifies during exercise or in hot environments. The degree of sweating varies from person to person, but 2 to 10 percent of patients regret having had the surgery, most frequently due to excessive compensatory sweating. As a result, some surgeons prefer to clamp the sympathetic trunk instead of severing or removing a segment to allow for the possibility of reversing the process if the compensatory sweating is disabling. However, there are no reports of successfully eliminating the sweating after removing the clamps, and reinnervation, which causes the original symptoms to return, occurs more frequently with this method.[60]

Detailed research has been done on the potential complications of

---

56 See, for example, A. Adair et al. (2005); C. Drott et al. (2002); R. Jeganathan et al. (2008); P. B. Licht et al. (2006); and NICE clinical guidelines (2014).
57 See K. Smidfelt and C. Drott (2011).
58 See T. A. Ojimba and A. E. Cameron (2004).
59 See C. H. Schick and T. Horbach (2003); and E. Jadresic et al. (2011).
60 See C. Suárez et al. (2005).

ETS,[61] including Horner's syndrome (1 percent); pneumothorax or pleural drainage (2 percent); intercostal neuritis, which I personally experienced (1 to 6 percent); sympathetic reinnervation with reappearance of symptoms up to one year after the operation (2 percent); and gustatory sweating when individuals eat certain foods (10 percent). Without being alarmist (after all, I benefited from the surgery), I should comment that the operation has been performed much less frequently in recent years in Sweden, a pioneer in the field, probably due to the public notoriety of a few patients who developed complications, and that in 2004 Taiwanese health authorities prohibited the procedure for those under age twenty.[62] My opinion is that, in all likelihood, when videothoracoscopic techniques simplified the procedure, many patients underwent surgery unnecessarily. This undoubtedly altered the risk/benefit ratio, with side effects becoming more heavily weighted; the surgery's reputation then came into question, resulting in the restrictions in Sweden and Taiwan. The restrictions underscore the need for health professionals, especially mental health specialists, to give due attention to blushing, to familiarize themselves with the patients' evaluation, to work closely with surgical teams, and to exhaust other psychological and pharmacological alternatives available in order to ensure that the surgery is used only as a last resort.

Since sympathectomy has long been used to treat facial blushing and hand sweating, and because biological studies indicate that the sympathetic nervous system regulates these symptoms in social phobia, it has been deemed ethical to extend studies of the possible effects of this surgery in SAD cases as well. Research available to date has been encouraging.[63] Our experience suggests that better results are attained with the sympathectomy when a psychiatric evaluation is done prior to the surgery. Of course, surgery is usually considered for patients with an incapacitating condition that has not responded to other types of treatment. While PB is a common denominator in all the cases described in the following chapters, every one of the individuals also suffered social anxiety to a significant degree, and most, if not all, met the current criteria for SAD.

---

61 See A. D. Burlan et al. (2000).

62 See details in www.wikipedia.org/wiki/Endoscopic_thoracic_sympathectomy.

63 See P. Pohjavaara and T. Telaranta (2005); and E. Jadresic et al. (2011).

Enrique Jadresic, MD

Finally, I would like to emphasize the importance of obtaining detailed informed consent from patients prior to the surgery. In our experience, and in that of other authors, a sympathectomy that is unsuccessful in treating PB can increase a patient's feelings of helplessness and depression, even in the absence of side effects. With unsuccessful surgery, the individual feels that he or she has tried everything and that there is no hope for a cure. It is important to analyze this possibility prior to surgery. In addition, experience shows that it is easier for patients to deal with poor surgical results when they receive psychiatric help. This also gives the patient and physician the option of considering, and ultimately beginning (or restoring, if it has been used previously), treatment with antidepressants, which, in addition to improving the patient's mood, can help lessen blushing, as we have seen.

Part Two

The Light at the End of the Tunnel

Chapter 6
Lucia D.

Mrs. Lucia D. was born in Santa Cruz, a small town in the Colchagua Valley, the heart of Chile's wine country. She is the fifth of six siblings, four of whom were living in the United States when we met. Like many other Chileans born in 1973, as a small child she became used to the fact that the mere mention of her birth year aroused all kinds of comments among her compatriots, but rarely indifference. After all, she came into the world in the same year that President Allende was overthrown in a military coup. But as time went by, she noticed that these comments were less frequent. *Memory can be very selective,* Lucia undoubtedly thought at some point.

Dr. Suárez had referred Lucia to me. She had made an appointment with him after watching a medical program on television during which he was mentioned in connection with surgical treatment for hyperhidrosis and blushing. He recommended that she come to me for an evaluation as to whether she was a good candidate for an endoscopic sympathectomy.

During our interview, Lucia told me she had been friendly and outgoing in school. "I volunteered for all the school programs," she said. She was also a good student. She first studied in a public school for girls, where she experienced no difficulty whatsoever. Two years before graduation, she transferred to a coed high school, where her life continued smoothly except for perhaps feeling slightly reserved due to the sudden proximity of boys. After finishing secondary school, she enrolled in a local technical institute, from which she graduated after five semesters with a degree as an agricultural technician.

I evaluated her in my office in Santiago quite some time back, in June

2005. She was thirty-two then, and she was happily married to a man one year older, a sociable fellow who worked in sales. They had two children, a daughter who was then eight and a son of about six. She told me that she had started working full time ten years before at a winery; it was then, as she recalled, that her blushing began. It occurred particularly "when I'm not ready," as she said. She noted that it happened when she was the focus of attention and when she was asked questions in public, especially if it was unexpected and she had to talk to someone who ranked above her in the company. Still, through hard work and determination, she had been able to have a fairly successful career. She had even been promoted to a position that included quality-control tasks that were normally performed by a college graduate, and she suspected that she could, over time, replace her boss (fortunately he was in agreement). However, she knew that her blushing limited her opportunities.

Lucia's search for help began with a visit to a psychiatrist. He prescribed alprazolam,[64] which she felt helped her to some extent. She later underwent psychotherapy with a psychologist but to no avail. Referring to the consequences of her blushing, she said, "I'm sick and tired of it"; after all, she'd been struggling with the problem for ten years. "I feel so stupid," she added. In other words, judging by the results of her job, she was outwardly successful but inwardly very frustrated. She was riddled with feelings of inadequacy, lacked self-confidence, and saw that she was likely to miss out on chances for advancement in her work.

A few days later, I e-mailed a report to Dr. Claudio Suárez with a basic medical and biographical report as well as the results of the clinical examination. I commented that Lucia's blushing had been very evident during the interview. In fact, despite the atmosphere of fellow-feeling that arose—that mutual understanding between two people who have suffered through the same problem—Lucia was clearly discomfited with her flaming cheeks. I asked her to fill out some questionnaires, which I told her I would have her complete once again after the surgery if she did have it.

I stated first in my report that I was surprised that the onset of the

---

64 Alprazolam belongs to the family of benzodiazepines. It is effective in treating anxiety, but it is used only for short periods of time, as it can cause dependence.

problem in her case had been somewhat later than it had been in most of the patients I had evaluated, whose symptoms tended to begin in puberty or adolescence. I then said that, in my opinion, Lucia suffered a great deal from the blushing. Last, and in light of her goal, which was clearly to lessen or eradicate the facial reddening, I concluded, "Mrs. Lucia D. suffers from pathological blushing without hyperhidrosis. She has a solid marriage and a basically healthy personality. She is a very good candidate for a T2 sympathectomy."

By that time, I had evaluated over fifty patients, and I felt more confident in giving my opinion, which I felt could be helpful. Not only was I familiar with the vicissitudes of the surgery as a treatment, but I also had continued to study the issue and had acquired more and more clinical experience with pathological blushing (PB) patients. In addition, as far as I knew, there were no other mental health professionals in the country working with the problem of blushing, either alone or with a surgical team, so it seemed logical for Dr. Suárez to call on me for help.

I did not hear from Lucia again until about ten months later, when I sent her an e-mail asking her if she had undergone the operation and, if she had, if it had been worthwhile. Two days later, I received the following e-mail message in return:

> Hello, Doctor.
>
> Thank you for writing to me. I have a lot to tell you, and I would have liked to go and see you, but there never seems to be enough time! I had the surgery on July 23, 2005, and the results were immediate.
>
> Concerning the operation itself, the doctor told me I recovered very quickly. I only took the pain medication he prescribed the first day after the surgery because I had no more pain after that. The worst was when I awoke after the surgery and felt chest pain (it felt as if my chest had caved in), but that only lasted for about twenty-four hours.
>
> I had the surgery on a Saturday. Nobody in my family knew what was going on except my husband, who had to stay with the two children, so I went to Santiago alone and returned the next day. All went well, thank God.

Back at work the following Monday, I could already see the effects of the surgery, and my life clearly began to change. I was still nervous in the situations that had always made me tense, but instead of blushing I began to sweat on my back and stomach. That was at first; I handle these situations much better now. I am much more confident with my ideas, and I can now speak up on issues without having to hold myself back. Before, I would begin to blush and couldn't defend my point of view.

I feel a great peace of mind, and I'm happy. I used to have headaches and felt a great deal of sadness or anger. Sometimes I thought I might develop some kind of head illness and that I would die or go crazy!! I would lie awake at night thinking, *Why is this happening to me?*

One of my fears was that my personality might change for the worse after the operation, that I might get carried away without the "brake" I have always had keeping me in check. I thought I might become aggressive or arrogant, but that hasn't happened (fortunately!!).

I don't sweat so much now, only when I do sports. In any case, it isn't excessive (to be more specific, my T-shirt doesn't get wet).

Since I know I'm not going to blush at just anything,[65] I now go into tense situations much more relaxed and calm. I laugh to myself sometimes about the change; it's incredible!! I never thought it would be so simple to do away with that torment of so many years!!

---

65 As was stated in chapter 5, endoscopic thoracic sympathectomy (ETS) decreases the intensity, frequency, and duration of facial blushing substantially, but it does not suppress it altogether (or at least it does not completely eliminate the sensation of blushing). Patients who are going to have surgery are informed of this fact. I have rarely heard patients report that their blushing has ceased entirely. In any case, we should not underestimate the possible significance of the expectation of complete blush suppression, since it helps patients face potential blush-inducing situations more calmly.

I am grateful to you and Dr. Suárez for working with this problem, since nobody knows or talks about it. More than an illness, people tend to associate it with personality problems. I think God must have put me in front of the TV screen just when Dr. Suárez's program was on. Otherwise I would still have the problem, and I would still be thinking there was no solution.

Well, Doctor, that is part of my story. If you would like more information, don't hesitate to write me; I'd be happy to tell you more!!

With a hug,
Lucia D.

I thanked Lucia for her testimony, of course. In addition, as I had told her during our interview, I asked her to respond to the same surveys that she had filled out when she was in my office, three well-known questionnaires that psychiatrists around the world use to quantify the degree of social anxiety a person feels in certain situations. They also measure the intensity of avoidance behavior, and one survey in particular quantifies the severity of the physiological symptoms associated with the anxiety.[66]

We have remained in contact sporadically over the years, which has enabled me to request, every now and then, that she answer these and other surveys by e-mail. The following graphs represent Lucia's pre- and postoperative scores on two of the questionnaires. Her responses nine months and then eighty months (almost seven years) after the endoscopic thoracic sympathectomy (ETS) show quantitatively the changes she experienced after the surgery.

Figure 6-1 shows a very significant decrease in the patient's level of social anxiety according to the Brief Social Phobia Scale. This decline not only remains steady over time but becomes even more marked.

---

66 The three questionnaires are the Liebowitz Social Anxiety Scale (LSAS), see M. R. Liebowitz (1987); the Brief Social Phobia Scale (BSPS), see J. R. T. Davidson et al. (1997); and the Social Phobia Inventory (SPIN), see K. M. Connor et al. (2000).

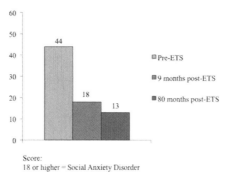

Score:
18 or higher = Social Anxiety Disorder

Figure 6-1. Change in Lucia's social anxiety levels following treatment with ETS (as measured by the Brief Social Phobia Scale).

Figure 6-2, in turn, shows a significant decrease in the level of social anxiety Lucia reported after the surgery, according to the Social Phobia Inventory, compared to when she first sought help. Whereas before the ETS she far exceeded the score needed for a diagnosis of social anxiety disorder (SAD), nine months after the surgical procedure her score was well below the minimum SAD diagnosis score of 19. Again, this decrease has lasted, and it is even more pronounced almost seven years later.

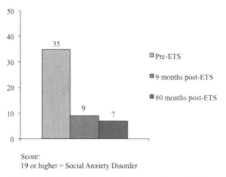

Score:
19 or higher = Social Anxiety Disorder

Figure 6-2. Change in Lucia's social anxiety levels after treatment with ETS (as measured by the Social Phobia Inventory).

We doctors like to quantify or monitor the decrease in symptoms as a result of treatment. In this respect, figure 6-3 shows that while Lucia categorized her facial reddening as "extreme" before the surgery, she responded "none" both times she was asked about her level of blushing after the operation.

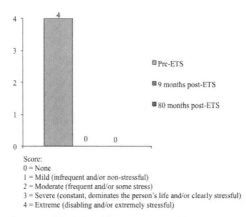

Score:
0 = None
1 = Mild (infrequent and/or non-stressful)
2 = Moderate (frequent and/or some stress)
3 = Severe (constant, dominates the person's life and/or clearly stressful)
4 = Extreme (disabling and/or extremely stressful)

Figure 6-3. Degree of facial reddening reported by Lucia when in contact with other people or when thinking of being with other people, before and after the ETS ("reddening" item on the Brief Social Phobia Scale).

In addition, Lucia has answered two other surveys over the years, one to evaluate compensatory sweating and the other to determine her degree of satisfaction with the surgery. Regarding the former, she has reported slight compensatory sweating[67] (fig. 6-4).

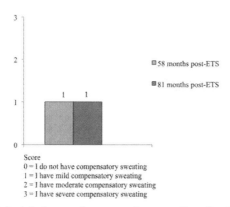

Score
0 = I do not have compensatory sweating
1 = I have mild compensatory sweating
2 = I have moderate compensatory sweating
3 = I have severe compensatory sweating

Figure 6-4. Lucia's degree of compensatory sweating after the surgery.

---

67 According to the standardized instrument used, slight compensatory sweating means, "I perspire a little when it is hot, when I exercise, or when I am under psychological stress. The perspiration does not run and I do not need to change clothes. The perspiring is tolerable and does not cause significant problems." See R. de M. Lyra et al. (2008).

Regarding Lucia's degree of satisfaction with the operation, on the two occasions when I have asked her opinion, she has selected "It helped a great deal" or "I am very satisfied" as the response that best represents her level of satisfaction.[68]

I was writing the first edition of *When Blushing Hurts* almost two years after Lucia D. had had her surgery. I called her at work one day to see how she was doing, and the person who answered the phone told me that Lucia had just given birth to her third child the day before and was therefore taking her well-deserved maternity leave. I did not know at the time how her job was going, but I was sure that she had her mind on other things that day. Some time later, I received the following message:

> Santa Cruz, April 2, 2007
> Dear Doctor,
>
> How are you coming on the book you were thinking of writing? When it's done I'll buy it and give it to my husband because, although he has always supported me in everything, he doesn't really understand how difficult this problem can be. After reading the book, he will finally be convinced of the necessity of the operation and how much it has helped me!! I'm sending you all of my energy to encourage you to finish the book; it will surely be an oasis in the middle of the desert for others like me!!
>
> Regards,
> Lucia D.

Soon, nine years will have passed since that cold winter day when she arrived, hopeful, at my office in the Providencia district of Santiago. I interviewed her in order to tell her and Claudio Suárez, as a psychiatrist but also as a patient with experience in the matter, whether ETS would be

---

68 The degree of satisfaction with the operation was determined with the same method as that used by P. Pohjavaara et al. (2003). To summarize, the evaluation includes the following items: degree of overall satisfaction, impact on job performance, impact on sentimental or romantic relationships, and impact on other social relationships primarily friendships). Because of space limitations, figure 6-4 reflects only Lucia's overall satisfaction with the surgery.

advisable in her case. We had a pleasant, prolonged conversation that day. Our paths have not crossed again, but I know that her parents are still alive; that she is happily married; and that her children are seventeen, fifteen, and six years old. She is still working at the winery, but only half-time. She is now the quality assurance supervisor, with five quality analysts working under her, and she works with people throughout the company, including the executives, on training matters. In addition, Lucia and her husband have started a new business, and she handles the administrative part. They have done quite well, and she is happy. Regarding the operation, she says, "It was and continues to be successful. For me, the blushing problem has been resolved."

We have been in contact only occasionally. Even so, we are bound by the ties that, due to a specific, shared circumstance, have made two people significant in each other's lives.

Chapter 7
Barbara F.

Barbara, who was born in 1972, lives in Santiago. Her father, a farmer, and her mother, a nurse, live in Talca, a town in southern Chile. The younger of two sisters, Barbara is a psychologist. She is married to an engineer, and they have two beautiful children. The older one has been slow in developing, a primary factor in her choosing not to work outside the home.

Although Barbara is the first one in her family to seek help for a propensity for excessive blushing, she is not the only one whose cheeks turn red at the slightest provocation. Her mother, now in her seventies, blushed so profusely as a child that many people called her "little apple." I do not know if it was a friendly nickname, if she disliked it, and if she ever considered the blushing a problem. But for Barbara, facial reddening has been troublesome for a long time. As she says,

> I remember having a tendency to blush easily since I was a small child and frequently being the butt of comments and jokes about it. Comments like, "Look, how sweet, she's blushing!" or "It looks like she's embarrassed," always bothered me to no end. It was so easy for me to blame and chastise myself for it! I never understood why people said these things or what the motive was behind their remarks. I certainly didn't find it amusing, if that's what they wanted. It only made me feel more embarrassed than I already was. I very rarely showed my anger; most of the

time I preferred to stay silent and hide my humiliation with
a fake smile, which made me feel even more ridiculous.

Clearly, those who make fun of someone who blushes seldom realize
the effects of their words. Low self-esteem looms like a shadow over those
who have suffered as the object of these jokes. As Barbara grew up and
faced the challenges of daily life, her demoralizing tendency to blush—
which most people make light of, sure that it is simply a problem of youth
that will disappear over time—never went away. Let's look at how she
experienced these symptoms and how things changed after her surgery:

> I don't know if the blushing got worse as I got older, but
> I feel that it began to cause problems in my life. I never
> seriously considered locking myself up in the house, but
> I certainly felt like it; I felt like just staying home. All
> it took for my face to go up in flames was to run into
> someone I knew at the supermarket or in the street. It
> was so embarrassing! Some things that happened were
> even funny. Of course now, after the operation, I see it
> all in a different light and it seems funny, but at the time
> I really suffered a great deal. At the end, right before the
> surgery, I was terribly depressed and full of anxiety. I saw
> my problem as practically an existential misfortune; it
> made me do things I didn't want to and kept me from
> doing other things that I wanted to achieve. There was a
> part of me that wanted to go out, meet people, laugh, be
> outgoing, give opinions, and ask questions. I just wanted
> to be happy, but this problem, this "accursed problem,"
> wouldn't let me.

In the paragraph above, as in other testimonies I have had the
opportunity to read, we see how what is presumably a minor symptom,
blushing in this case, can erode not only self-esteem but also the will and
desire to live. Thus Barbara spoke of an existential misfortune.

Also, Barbara's last statement about what she wanted, which was to
"embrace the world" as we described it metaphorically earlier, demonstrates

how pathological blushing (PB) works as a kind of "brake" in many patients' lives. A phenomenon we frequently see is that individuals experience the blushing as something that does not live inside of them, so to speak, but rather is imposed on them from the outside. Thus they speak of a brake holding them back, of a glass wall cutting them off, and of opposing forces struggling against one another. In other words, many patients say they feel like a puzzle or a mosaic whose pieces do not fit. On the one hand, they perceive an expansive, centrifugal nature inside of themselves that drives them to be gregarious and reach out to others, while on the other hand there is this "accursed" invisible wall that separates them from the world and that they anxiously seek to break through.[69]

Let's continue with Barbara's story:

> I began to want to withdraw from people, hoping not to see anyone, to disappear, run away … until one day I just couldn't take it anymore after what was frankly an awful, humiliating experience (I'm not exaggerating) at the grocery store. I went in tears back to the car, where my husband was waiting for me. I remember that he had no idea what was going on; I had never told him or anyone else of the bondage in which I was living. Maybe he suspected something; I suppose he did, but it never occurred to me to tell him something so intimate, so painful, and so degrading. Other people see it as something quirky that can be controlled, and they think that you're probably

---

69 As a doctor, I find it interesting to contrast this phenomenon with what occurs in depression, where, in general, patients consider the depressive "darkness" to be something that is inside of them, a part of their innermost selves, rather than something that has come to them from the outside. Also, my experience with patients who undergo surgery for blushing takes me back to my days at medical school, when I tended to find the surgery patients that I saw much less "ill," as it were, or with a pathology that was much more clearly confined, than what I observed in internal medicine patients. Surgery patients tended to consider what was happening to them as external, alien to them in a sense, and it did not affect them in such a global way (it is the gallbladder that is ill, not the patient, so to speak). Likewise, when I see PB patients, it still surprises me that they give the impression of being basically healthy (like the patients I saw in surgery) despite their intense suffering.

exaggerating, but it's something you have to go through to understand. That was when my husband told me that a few years before he had read in a magazine or a newspaper about an operation that took care of the problem. I looked on the Internet and was amazed to discover that there was such an operation, and that they even did it in Chile. I confess that if they had been doing it in China, I would have gone to China. I was in a really, really bad way back then; I was tired, exhausted. There were certain blushing situations that had a logical explanation, but others that were simply ludicrous.

When I evaluated Barbara in June 2005, it seemed to me that she was a good candidate for endoscopic thoracic sympathectomy (ETS). I said as much to her and to Dr. Claudio Suárez, and a few weeks later, Barbara went into the operating room. She was out in an hour; the surgery had gone smoothly.

Just as I had been when I first assessed a patient for a possible ETS, Barbara was in the throes of anxiety when she went to see Dr. Suárez for her first postoperative checkup. She tells of her experience:

Dr. Suárez and I had agreed to meet after the operation, and I confess that I was terrified. Had it been successful? What if I was one of those patients that do not respond well? It couldn't be all that wonderful! I couldn't imagine my life without this problem. What would life, my life, be like without blushing, without having to be always running away and hiding? I don't know if I turned red that day; I don't remember anymore. But I can say that my life did change, and for the better, after the operation.

Let's see exactly what happened and how Barbara evaluated the results of the surgery twelve months later:

I don't mind anymore when I walk down the street and run into an acquaintance, attend meetings at my children's school, share my opinion with a group, when someone draws attention to me, or when someone calls my name and/or makes a comment about me in public. It has to be a really, truly horrible situation for me to feel that I'm beginning to blush. What I have felt is a sort of pressure in my face, like an electric current that comes and then fades away. Because of all these changes, I find myself several times a day thanking God and being grateful to the doctor who performed the surgery and to my husband for all of their help and support because that is what the surgery has been for me: a *huge help*. I don't really even remember any of the possibly unpleasant side effects I was told I might have; the compensatory sweating, for example. My body, back, and legs sweat a little more, but not enough to be a problem. Maybe I never did perspire much; I don't know, but I would really be exaggerating if I said that it was a concern for me now. I have never been aware of having a damp blouse or pants, and no one has ever said anything to me about it.

Suddenly, situations that most people take for granted (walking anxiety-free down the street, hearing one's name without feeling one's cheeks flush crimson) become a new and wonderful "discovery" for the blushing patient who has had successful surgery. Regarding compensatory sweating, judging from her testimony one year after the surgery, this has not been a significant problem for Barbara. However, on two subsequent occasions she answered questionnaires on this aspect, and on both she reported a certain degree of discomfort. Both at fifty-eight months and at eighty-one months after the surgery (almost five and almost seven years later), she chose option 3 ("have moderate compensatory sweating") among four options of increasing severity.[70]

Looking back on her case with the perspective of time, I would venture

---

70 According to the instrument used, moderate compensatory sweating means, "I perspire moderately when it is hot, when I exercise, or when I am under psychological stress. Perspiration droplets form and run, but I do not need to change clothes. Although it is uncomfortable, it is not something that embarrasses me."

to say that Barbara has become not only a happier person but also a wiser one. This is evident in the few lines she sent me some years ago:

> Finally, I would like to say that at first it's hard to get used to living without this problem, to get used to the idea that this "silly blushing" is no longer with you wherever you go; at least that's what happened to me. But it's important not to be impatient because the results and peace of mind come gradually over time. There comes a time when the problem, silently and surprisingly, ceases to be the focus of your life.[71] However, it's very important to have realistic expectations about the operation in that you shouldn't think that after the surgery you'll become a different person, a sort of "king" (or queen) of assertiveness and self-confidence at any and all times. I don't believe that is possible, much less an ideal. What I do believe, and I think it is good and healthy, is in trying to figure out the message behind the problem either before or after the surgery. It is a message that can tell us a lot about ourselves, our personal characteristics, and our nature; messages that our body sends us, and, through our body, alert us to our problem or limitation. As a well-known and highly respected Chilean psychiatrist, Adriana Schnake, said, "We generally become angry at and struggle with that part

---

71 I do not believe it would be an exaggeration to say that most of my PB patients' lives revolve around the problem of blushing. Barbara tells us that if the operation had been available only in China, she would have gone there for it. I have heard similar comments several times, evidence of the extremes to which people are willing to go to find a solution. For the same reason, I am amazed to see that at some point after the operation, patients' attention ceases to be focused on facial reddening. The various stimuli that bring on blushing or anticipatory anxiety (e.g., going out or speaking in public) finally take on their true dimensions for these individuals. In other words, blushing is now a possibility rather than the focal point of psychological experience. For example, I know of one case, a young man who did not even have a girlfriend and yet agonized over the possibility of blushing on his wedding day. I suspect that his fears have dissipated if he has had the surgery.

of our body that shows us our limitation or bothers us in some way, and, because of that, we do not talk to it, much less listen to it." Therefore, the "invitation," I would dare to say, is to take advantage of this opportunity, believe me, this great chance that our dearly beloved blushing gives us to explore it, with warmth and acceptance, trying to understand it and get a little closer to it and, as a result, to our true being.

For those who like quantification, I can say that over the years I have asked Barbara to answer the same surveys on degree of satisfaction with the surgery that Lucia answered in the previous chapter. On a scale of 1 to 5, in order of increasing satisfaction, twenty-four months postoperation she chose option 5 ("it was very helpful/very satisfied"), and at eighty-one months (almost seven years after the surgery) she answered with option 4 ("it was quite helpful/quite satisfied"). Barbara's recent statement, almost nine years after the treatment she chose, only confirms this positive opinion:

Santiago, January 1, 2014
Hello, Doctor,

I have been great these last two years. I blush, but within normal parameters. I can go anywhere, I can run into people, raise my hand to give my opinion, and get involved in arguments without "suffocating." I have a very positive evaluation of the operation and, if I were to experience what I went through before, or even a fraction of it, I would have the surgery again. It is one of those before and after moments in my life.

Regards,
Barbara

Chapter 8
Benjamin S.

Benjamin believed that his life began to change when he submitted the word "blushing" to a Google search (the term was actually *rubor facial*; Benjamin is a native Spanish speaker). Until then, he had lived almost a third of his thirty-four years feeling as if he were adrift in a quest for the solution to what he considered his main problem, a solution that had never materialized. He still lives in Aysen, in the far south of Chile, where he works in the salmon industry. His short-lived marriage lasted only a year due, in part, to his work schedule.

"You see, I work twenty days straight at the salmon farm, and then I have ten days off at home in Puerto Montt. No woman can take that," he explained, settling into his chair across from me at my office. "It's not an easy life for a wife."

I pointed out that he did not seem troubled. He admitted that he was not and then added, "If I knew that I wasn't ever going to blush, I would always be as calm as I am talking with you right now."

He appeared serene and hopeful, probably influenced (as he admitted in a written testimony he sent to me several months later) by a sympathectomy experience he had heard firsthand and by learning of the possibility of putting an end to his years of torment.

The following is a transcription of part of Benjamin's vivid account of his experiences prior to the surgery:

> About *fifteen* years ago, I began to feel an unpleasant blush
> come over my face in varying degrees under different social

circumstances. At first I tried to ignore it and not consider it a problem, but the intensity and frequency of blushing forced me to seek medical help. I went to several doctors during those years (about six), but since their diagnoses were not correct, the treatments were not effective, and my problem continued. I remember their recommending that I expose myself to the situations that caused the blushing; supposedly, if I faced the circumstances time and again, the symptoms would eventually begin to subside. Of course, this never occurred, and, besides, the whole situation was virtually torture for me. Since I quit the treatments, considering them ineffective, I was always left with a twinge of doubt: what would happen if I actually finished a course of treatment recommended by a doctor? So I embarked on four years of therapy (four years!!). I was diagnosed with social phobia, which I have, of course, and was given antidepressants and anxiolytics. But since, once again, the effects rather than the cause itself were being treated, my condition didn't improve significantly. I suppose the antidepressants helped me maintain a certain level of optimism, but I honestly never felt that different, and the blushing continued.

Let's pay close attention to what Benjamin said next:

I admit that it wasn't easy to identify the problem. True, it was obvious that I blushed easily, but I attributed it to a myriad of other reasons. I questioned my capacity for facing challenges and my mental toughness. I didn't know that blushing was a problem in itself and, assuming it was caused by a mental problem of some kind, I plunged enthusiastically into a course of therapy and drug treatment, hoping to find the solution there. Nothing helped, and I became very frustrated.

"But what exactly is blushing? What do you feel?" Benjamin wondered about blushing. He answered the question himself:

It's fear … fear of blushing and of others seeing my face looking like a tomato; embarrassment that it's happened again, that I can't control it, that it's betrayed me yet again. What else do you feel? Outright humiliation and a sense of inferiority that gradually drags you down, almost to depression, because you've tried everything and nothing helps. Of course, the effects continue as long as you don't deal with the root cause, so then you have to deal with the enormous psychological exhaustion too, since your mind is always struggling to keep the symptoms from appearing. Your whole life seems to get darker and darker with these frequent, intense blushing episodes until you can't stand it anymore and all you want to do is stay home and never go anywhere. Every time you go out is pure torture. There's always a chance of another humiliation because you feel that you don't control it, but that it controls you. You begin to doubt yourself in every way, and the only thing you want is to talk to someone without blushing. I even stopped using the word *red*, stopped thinking it or looking at red objects; I tried to avoid the color completely.

He then went on and described his efforts to overcome his blushing:

I tried mental strategies for not turning red: concentrating only on the moment, on my breathing, etc. I tried a lot of alternative spiritual reading and practices, such as Reiki and meditation, looking for a solution that, of course, never appeared. You tend to hide, stay out of sight, cover up, so that other people don't see what's happening. I wear a beard, I wear a hat whenever I can, and I always have my sunglasses; I withdraw and constantly avoid social contact. I developed a social phobia, an anticipatory anxiety about blushing. As you can see, it's not a pleasant state to be in. I suffer because if I go out into the "world" I'm liable to blush, and if I don't, I end up locked up inside the four walls of my house. I'm trapped either way. If you're having a really hard time and there's nowhere to turn, one alternative is drinking. Of course, alcohol abuse is just adding another problem. Still, it has sometimes been my salvation, and I suppose there must be a lot of alcoholics who started drinking because of pathological blushing.[72]

Benjamin talked about his years of mortification, his most difficult times. He also mentioned the numerous personal disguises and amulets that have allowed him—and others—to "survive" this labyrinth with no way out. Listening to him in my office or reading his testimony was like looking at myself in a mirror. I identified so closely with his suffering that, having recently read that it is easy to provoke a blush in a person who blushes readily simply by saying that he or she is already red, I was not capable of testing it on him. When I interview patients and we get to this point, it is not just ethical reservations that make me abandon my usual cerebral attitude and avoid deliberately inducing a blush; it is simple human solidarity, compassion, or unavoidable complicity, if you will, with a fellow sufferer. I welcome a patient's blushing in my presence, but it is a subtle rather than overt welcome. If, however, the person's cheeks never turn crimson, I do not force it, preferring rather to trust my patient's word. But let's let Benjamin continue:

My worst years were at college. I remember that for a long time I would go into the classroom just a few seconds before the class started and leave immediately afterward, struggling the whole time to keep the blushing at bay.[73]

---

72 Social anxiety disorder (SAD) and/or pathological blushing (PB) patients frequently abuse substances, especially alcohol, and many alcoholics report preexisting social anxiety. Indeed, of all patients with social anxiety disorders, social phobics are those most likely to abuse alcohol.

73 What Benjamin describes reminds me of my own experience. While at the university, I had my own father as a professor (of psychiatry, to be precise) for a time. Theoretically, his classes started at 2:30 p.m., but he usually arrived five to ten minutes late. Those few minutes, when generally the entire class—including me—was sitting in the room waiting for him to arrive, were torture for me: My classmates would begin to make friendly but predictable jokes ("it must have been a good nap," "must be having a great lunch," etc.). I did not mind the jokes at all—I even thought they were funny—but I *was* disturbed by

My deep anxiety obviously compromised my intellectual abilities, so I had to deal not only with blushing but also with poor grades. Despite all the difficulties brought on by blushing and contrary to what one might expect, I managed to earn two degrees, get married, and find a good job in my profession, but it was all at the cost of a tremendous internal struggle and by strictly limiting my social activities. I have almost come to believe that this is normal.

I have had to develop an incredibly thick skin because I all too frequently suffer humiliations and then have to face the same people the next day as if nothing has happened (I think that you can only understand this fully if you've experienced it). I have forgotten what it is to enjoy social activities, since the fear of blushing is always with me and takes over my mind, although I try to avoid it. I have almost forgotten how to be happy and have got used to a very dreary life. It has also affected the professional and sentimental sides of my life.[74]

What other strategies do you use to survive? Avoidance, or automatically rejecting any social activity that might trigger the problem. You then realize that since all social activities are potential blushing episodes, there are very few places left where you will feel comfortable. Everyday activities like going to class, riding the city bus, or going shopping are a torture that ends only when you

---

the heightened state of vigilance they provoked in me as well as by the thought that, once again, my physiological hypersensitivity would give me away in front of my classmates. 74 Another patient, a bank teller, is a case in point for the professional limitations sometimes experienced by individuals with PB. This woman's job performance improved so radically after her endoscopic thoracic sympathectomy (ETS) that she was soon promoted to account executive. She then did so well in that position that a year after the surgery she had garnered all that year's performance awards. So dramatic was the change that the bank management started an investigation to see why such an exceptional employee had not been promoted earlier.

go to sleep, and not really even then since you know that the next day will be more of the same.[75]

The Light at the End of the Tunnel

In a way, as time goes by you learn to handle the blushing, or maybe you get used to it. It's true that there are days and moments when everything's not so bad, but still it's a draining, exhausting, depressing problem.

Not long ago I did a Google search with the word "blushing" [again, the term actually searched was *rubor facial*] and found a number of pages, including Dr. Claudio Suárez's, which discusses how this problem has its roots in the sympathetic nervous system and that a surgical procedure can correct it. Imagine the joy I felt! However, it didn't last long since I also read the opinions of people who regretted having had the operation, mostly because of a side effect known as compensatory sweating: Because perspiration no longer occurs on the face, armpits, or hands, depending on each case, other parts of the body sweat more heavily. My fears finally dissipated when I heard firsthand the experience of someone who had had a sympathectomy, and the possibility of ending years of suffering allows me to imagine a quality of life that I never dreamed possible. Finally, I'd like to say that this isn't shyness or the blushing of a teenager who's been caught doing something he shouldn't, and it's not something that can be handled through willpower or effort. It's pathological. I don't want to sound like it's the worst thing that can happen to someone, but I don't want it to be minimized or belittled, either, or brushed off as

---

75 I would like to point out another observation Benjamin made in the interview that illustrates the discrepancy that frequently exists between PB patients' self-perception and how others see them. He said, "People think I am distant and cold ... it's because I'm protecting myself." This is a good example of how, in psychology, appearances can be deceiving.

insignificant. I'm giving my testimony because if it gets published, I want people who read it and identify with it to be able to look for a concrete solution. I'm not playing the victim; I'm just describing my life as a pathological blusher as objectively as I can. Now, less than a month before the surgery, I'm trusting God that it will all turn out right.

Benjamin was one of the few patients who did not come alone to my office. He came with his father, Adrian, a friendly man of around sixty who had taken early retirement. I asked him to come in, and he took part in the conversation:

"I still blush even today. I always got blamed for everything in school. I turned red even if I hadn't done anything wrong, and my classmates would say, 'Adrian did it.' I had a hard time, of course."[76]

Adrian said that he had always told Benjamin that blushing was normal, but that he did notice his son had almost no social life and that when he did go out, it was always at night.

Benjamin underwent surgery at the end of January 2006. In March 2007, he gave me his opinion of his therapeutic process:

> I made the decision to have the surgery after seeing a specialist in the field who had also had the same operation. It gave me much more confidence and peace of mind to know that a serious health professional had had a successful operation. The procedure itself was done with general anesthesia, and I must confess that the recovery was difficult. The first *twelve* hours were the worst, when

---

76 It is common during interviews with PB patients or their relatives to find that there are immediate family members with the same disorder, although the cases are not always as intense. An extreme example of this is a family that I evaluated from the north of Chile. After one of the sisters had surgery and was very satisfied with the outcome, another sister followed suit, and then another, and another. Finally, all five siblings (four sisters and a brother) underwent surgery to decrease excessive blushing. They were all very satisfied with the results, which are documented in written testimonies and in psychometric evaluations. Surprisingly (or perhaps not), in the next few days I will evaluate the mother of these patients; she is anxious to look into the option of surgery after seeing the changes in her children's lives.

I had a great deal of chest pain. But the pain gradually disappeared, and I was able to leave the hospital the next day with just slight discomfort.

I am quite satisfied with the results of the surgery. The objective was to eliminate the blushing and, while I have turned red a couple of times, I feel that the problem has decreased noticeably in frequency and intensity. Besides, because of this, my level of anxiety is also considerably lower since I no longer blush in the situations that I used to. I have become more confident and can live my life with a lot less stress. I'm thankful that I no longer have to be always thinking how I'm going to keep from blushing or avoiding people. In any case, it is a gradual process rather than an immediate change from one day to the next, especially for someone who has gotten used to a certain lifestyle. The change comes gradually and you have to overcome deeply ingrained behavior patterns, but it's been worth the effort, especially now that I have the resources to do it.

I haven't stopped blushing completely, but it is now to a degree that I find satisfactory. If I had to have the operation again with the same results, I'd do it without a second thought.

I have two side effects: compensatory sweating (I perspire a great deal on my chest and back) and dry hands. I have to be careful about wearing heavy clothes in order to not get them damp. It is very visible and can be a problem, but of course no worse than the blushing. Having dry hands is not usually noticeable, and it doesn't bother me.

Finally, I would like to say that having found a solution to my problem was, truly, like finding water in the desert or an island in the middle of the ocean. Discovering that there was a physiological cause let me stop thinking I was crazy and looking everywhere for improbable solutions. In short, it's been a great discovery.

My final recommendation to someone who identifies with this is: have the surgery.

Next, a look at Benjamin's pre- and postoperative questionnaires shows the changes he had undergone, first at four months and then at seventy-four months (six years), after the endoscopic thoracic sympathectomy (ETS).

Figure 8-1 shows that the Brief Social Phobia Scale identified Benjamin as a social anxiety disorder (SAD) patient prior to the surgery. Four months afterward, he no longer met the criteria for that diagnosis. Six years later, however, his score once again fell within the social phobia diagnosis.

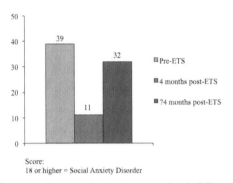

Figure 8-1. Change in Benjamin's social anxiety levels following treatment with ETS (as measured by the Brief Social Phobia Scale).

Likewise, figure 8-2 shows that, while Benjamin's score in the Social Phobia Inventory prior to the surgery identified him as a social phobia sufferer, the postoperative questionnaire results, at four months, did not support this diagnosis. But again, six years later he was back within the social phobia range.

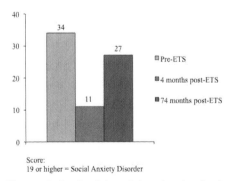

Figure 8-2. Changes in Benjamin's social anxiety levels after treatment with ETS (as measured by the Social Phobia Inventory).

In quantifying the blushing symptom, figure 8-3 shows that while Benjamin evaluated his blushing as "severe" before the surgery, he described it as "slight" when asked four months after the operation. However, six years later he once again considered his blushing to be "severe."

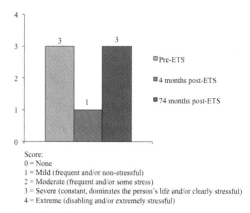

Score:
0 = None
1 = Mild (frequent and/or non-stressful)
2 = Moderate (frequent and/or some stress)
3 = Severe (constant, dominates the person's life and/or clearly stressful)
4 = Extreme (disabling and/or extremely stressful)

Figure 8-3. Degree of facial reddening reported by Benjamin when in situations involving contact with other people or when thinking about such a situation, before and after ETS.

When I sent Benjamin a questionnaire by e-mail ten months after the ETS to quantify his overall level of satisfaction with the operation, he responded immediately, as usual. On a scale of 1 to 5, in order of increasing satisfaction, the response that best described his experience was number 4, which meant "quite helpful" or "I'm satisfied." Six years later, however, he chose option 3 (meaning "somewhat helpful").

Benjamin's surgery was eight years ago. After seventeen months, I mentioned the possibility of meeting for a psychiatric checkup after the operation, but it was not necessary; our written exchanges and the successful outcome of the surgery seemed to suffice. The following lines reflect his perceptions of the results of the operation at that time:

> [E]verything turned out well. I was told I might suffer compensatory sweating, which I do, and it is worse than I expected. Still, I'm happy with my decision and very satisfied with the results since the symptoms I had before have not returned ... As to the psychiatric checkup, to be quite honest, I feel that I now have the resources to go on

with my life. My goals are very clear, and I feel peace of mind where before I felt only anxiety.

But enthusiasm sometimes wanes over time. Two years ago, Benjamin told me that he felt that the operation had not had the results he had hoped for. Still, he expressed satisfaction with his life in a message he sent me a few days ago:

I'm fine, and my family is too, thank you. I have not continued with any kind of treatment; in fact, I consider it a real achievement to have stayed away from any kind of medications. I have come up with strategies that help me feel comfortable and carry out my day-to-day activities without anxiety. Overall, I have a pleasant life and, although there are still challenges, they are more of a motivation than a problem. My daughters and my wife are a great help as well. I read the testimonies that you sent me, and it touches me deeply to see how a human being can find peace and overcome his fears ... We know that this is not a matter of life and death, but it is very disabling. It's a pleasure to be in touch with you again; I wish you lots of success. And thank you for your good wishes. May 2014 be a great year for you and your family!

Chapter 9
Martin P.

I met Martin eight years ago, when he was a junior in high school. He was the fourth of five children, and his family lived in a well-to-do Santiago neighborhood. When he came to see me with his parents, he told me that he had been having trouble with sweaty hands during the previous two or three years.

"It's very limiting in that I can't shake hands when greeting people."

This, of course, was no surprise to me.

He then commented that he had always had a tendency to blush profusely and that it had even intensified over the last few months.

The distress in his crimson face said it all. He noted that the problem was getting worse and was affecting his social relationships, self-esteem, moods, and school grades. When we were alone, he added that an older brother frequently made fun of him, something that his parents, particularly his father, made light of.

He described himself as having been "mischievous and funny" as a child. In answer to a question of mine, he responded, "I used to have a lot more personality, but I'm losing it. It's like a light going off. And I'm losing interest in school. I used to get better grades."

He attributed these changes to the symptoms he had described, which, he acknowledged, were generally brought on by emotional stimuli.

When I talked to Martin's parents alone, his mother was understanding. She said, "I've found him in tears, and he's never been one much given to crying." She added, "He doesn't want to go to Mass in order to avoid having to give the handshake of peace."

Martin's father was somewhat indifferent. "I don't know if it's the hand sweating, the blushing, or a teenage crisis, but I do know that it's causing problems in the family, poisoning the atmosphere. You can see his long face from a hundred yards away."

Sometimes when Martin had complained of blushing, his father had responded, "Don't complain to me; the same thing happens to me!"

Martin's parents had certainly noticed that he was moody, that he was going out less, and that he "didn't have energy to do anything." He was no longer the happy, outgoing kid they knew, who loved to mimic others.

When I explained to them that their son was suffering greatly and that the psychological consequences of palmar hyperhidrosis and pathological blushing (PB) could be serious, both parents' attitudes changed.

Martin had been treated unsuccessfully by several dermatologists, including six sessions of iontophoresis.[77] His mother, hopeful after talking with a friend whose daughter had had an endoscopic thoracic sympathectomy (ETS), was looking into the possibility of the surgery. One of the dermatologists, whom she had asked about the operation, had told her that Martin's problem would eventually subside. If it were his son, he would not have the surgery.

My response was that, considering my own experience with the problem and the surgery, if Martin were my son, I would not rule out having the operation. In my medical evaluation, I stated,

> To sum up, the patient presents palmar hyperhidrosis and PB, as well as depression.[78] He would very likely benefit from a sympathectomy. Although antidepressants could

77 Iontophoresis is an electricity-based technique and one that is frequently used to treat hyperhidrosis. It enables certain medications to be delivered through the skin so that they can take effect without having to pass through the digestive system or be administered in an injection.

78 I should point out that while in my first reports I explicitly stated when a patient clearly had social anxiety, or SAD, over time I began to omit the reference to social anxiety or avoidance symptoms. It is not that the symptoms were not present, but rather that they were found as a matter of course. Thus, implicit in an affirmation that a patient was a good candidate for a sympathectomy was the fact that he or she had SAD or significant anxiety symptoms.

be considered (a psychometric evaluation corroborated the diagnosis of depression), I inform the parents that SSRIs can increase sweating.[79] My prognosis is that if this boy has the surgery, he will undergo a remarkable mood change.

I did not hear from Martin again until eight months later. I learned through e-mail that the antidepressants had not been necessary. He had had the surgery and, according to the questionnaires he returned to me, he felt that the ETS had been "somewhat helpful." His mother, who was more emphatic, sent me the following message:

> Dear Enrique,
>
> I'm so sorry for not writing sooner. I assume that Martin sent the responses to the questionnaires. I have seen a radical change in his personality. He's much more self-confident and has a lot of friends. He's nicer, happier, and more relaxed and responsible. The operation was a success in every way. Martin is a whole new person. *Thank you so much for everything!*

I have attempted to contact Martin or his mother in recent years but to no avail. I hope that he is a happy, fulfilled young man. Looking back at his case with the perspective of eight years, I believe that his operation was somewhat hasty and that he should perhaps have first tried other psychological or pharmacological treatments. As young people are more adept at learning, cognitive-behavioral psychotherapy is a good option in these cases. Unfortunately, it is still very difficult in many countries to find therapists trained in the specific techniques used to treat these patients.

---

79 Since selective serotonin reuptake inhibitors (SSRIs) are known for increasing perspiration, for a time I was reluctant to prescribe this type of medication for patients who suffered from hyperhidrosis in addition to PB. However, in recent years I have frequently heard patients whom I have treated with SSRIs say that they notice a slightly increased tendency to perspire overall, but they also note a decrease in perspiration due to stress, the kind that disturbs them the most.

Chapter 10
Monica G., Sebastian L., and Camila V.

Monica, Sebastian, and Camila all have the same problem. They all underwent endoscopic thoracic sympathectomy (ETS) procedures searching for a solution to their tendency to blush excessively, and they developed, like many other patients, compensatory sweating. Let's take a look at a few aspects of their personal stories to learn how each one has experienced this side effect.

I met Monica nine years ago. She was married with two children, and she had worked for over twenty years as an administrative assistant in a laboratory. A dermatologist who had diagnosed her with rosacea had referred her to the thoracic surgeon. Before that, she had seen a psychiatrist for her shyness, which, she remembered, dated back to adolescence. *What happened to my other personality?* she often wondered, since she had been outgoing and gregarious as a child. She associated the personality change with the blushing. She had even undergone hypnosis to try to control it, but it had been unsuccessful.

She had not had a happy marriage. Her husband, an industrial worker, drank heavily, liked to go out with friends, and was well on his way to becoming a compulsive gambler. "The family has never been very important to him," she said. Now, when I interviewed Monica at the request of the surgeon, she seemed anxious to me. One of her comments was, "I know that if it gets hot I'm going to turn red. I can't control my nervous system!"

In my report, I wrote,

> Monica suffers from an anxiety disorder. She also presents
> with neck blushing and, to a lesser degree, facial blushing
> in the form of "splotches" associated primarily with high
> temperatures. I explained to her that she is not a good
> candidate for surgery, but I offered her the possibility of
> psychopharmacological treatment, which she accepted.

Although some months later she reported having less anxiety, the
selective serotonin reuptake inhibitor (SSRI) she was taking had no effect
on her blushing. A year later, she wrote to me to say that she had undergone
a T2 sympathectomy, and after that I did not hear from her for some time.

One summer almost four years later when I was doing a follow-up on
my patients, I received an e-mail from her:

> I'm Monica G. Do you remember me? Doctor, I have to
> be frank: the compensatory sweating is driving me crazy.
> I'm wet day and night, and it has become unbearable. I
> should be wearing light summer clothes in hot weather,
> but instead I have to wear an undershirt or a sweater to
> keep my wet clothing from being so noticeable. I can't
> even sit down on the bus or the subway because the heat
> is unbearable, and if I do, my clothes get all wet and stick
> to my body. I was really hopeful when I had the surgery,
> but I never imagined that I would perspire to this extent.

The compensatory sweating did not diminish over time. This is
Monica's opinion three years later:

> The perspiration continues to be a huge problem. I have
> to shower and change clothes more than once a day.
> My clothes stick to my body and itch, which is really
> unpleasant. If it were only on one part of my body it would
> be more tolerable, but I sweat on my back, abdomen, and

legs. All day long, I've got a drop of sweat (many drops) running down as if it were a faucet dripping and dripping.

Later, she continued:

About two years ago I went to see the surgeon about it, and he gave me oxybutynin[80] to help with the perspiring. I took it for a while, but the perspiration didn't decrease. It just made my mouth really dry and pasty; it was even hard to talk, so I quit taking it.

She added:

The perspiration increases considerably when I have a hot drink, ride on the bus or subway, or when I'm in an enclosed place. It's like I'm in a sauna. When I remember that I didn't even sweat under my arms before the surgery, I become furious with myself. Can I ask you the million-dollar question, Doctor? Is there a solution to this problem? Can the sympathetic nerve be reattached or restored?[81] Forgive me for going on like this, but I spend practically eight months out of the year struggling with the problem. It's only four months, maybe a little more, that I'm fine, without sweating excessively. You can understand that this situation separates me from the world around me. Now I have two problems: blushing (it's less intense, but I do still blush) and being constantly wet.

Surprisingly, despite the fact that the compensatory sweating had become a daily drama for her, when she answered a questionnaire for me

---

80 Oxybutynin is derived from botulinum toxin. It belongs to a group of medications called anticholinergics that decrease sweating. Many patients on oxybutynin eventually stop taking it due to its side effects, mainly dry mouth.
81 While there are anecdotal reports of surgeries reversing the effects of the ETS, they are not procedures supported by scientific evidence.

seven years later, she said she did not regret having the surgery and that it had been "somewhat helpful."

Sebastian was a sixteen-year-old high school student when the thoracic surgeon asked me to evaluate him eight years ago. He seemed to me to be a talented boy with a great deal of potential. He told me he blushed in many day-to-day situations: whenever he heard his name mentioned, when he got on a city bus, if someone on the street asked him the time, or when he was dealing with someone of the opposite sex. He avoided going out in the daytime ("It's easier for me to get together with girls at night," he explained), and he felt misunderstood. "My mother says I don't love myself," he says, and "My parents sometimes think my problem is ridiculous." I told the surgeon that Sebastian suffered from pathological blushing (PB) and that he would very likely benefit from a sympathectomy. I added, however, that he had agreed to try first with medications and that he would come back to see me in four months.

As it turned out, I did not see him again. However, three years later I received the following e-mail:

> Doctor Enrique,
>
> I am Sebastian L. I went once to your office because I was having difficulty with the problem of turning red. Well, I graduated from high school and, with the support of my family, I decided to have the surgery at the beginning of this year so that I could start college without blushing. Everything has gone well at the "U," and I've met a lot of people. But the fact that I've been able to be more outgoing has brought with it another "problem": There are a lot of girls who would like to go out with me, but I'm afraid to date and then want to start something more serious because of how I sweat. I'm worried about what they might say, and I'm worried that they might find it disgusting. That really bothers me. Knowing that you had the surgery too, and that you know about the problem, I thought I'd tell you about it to see if you could give me some advice.

I tried to help Sebastian and give him some guidance. We exchanged a few messages, but I soon lost track of him again. I do not know how he is or how he would rate the operation now.

Certainly, although messages such as these from Monica and Sebastian are not common, their words are powerful and cannot leave us indifferent. They show that we are still far from finding a satisfactory treatment for PB. In addition, they require that we be even more emphatic in stressing to our patients that the surgery involves risks and may cause permanent side effects and, therefore, must—necessarily—be considered a treatment option only for extreme cases.

I met Camila when she was thirty-two years old. She had been married for ten years, and she worked in a bank. Since she had not been able to have a baby, she and her husband were thinking of adopting a child. She told me that as a child she had always been a leader; in fact, she had been president of her eighth-grade class. As a teen, she began to turn red very easily, something that disturbed her greatly, especially, she said, because it also made it difficult for her to think clearly. She blushed when she was the center of attention, when she had to speak in public, or if someone played a joke on her or gave her a compliment. Her coworkers knew that she blushed easily, and those closest to her tried to "protect" her from exposure to these types of situations. She said that sessions with a psychologist had been helpful, but that she still blushed. She was taking three self-prescribed propranolol tablets a day. Her palms also sweated profusely when she was under stress, and she shrank from giving the handshake of peace when she went to Mass. As time passed, she had become more of a loner. "It's a kind of self-defense," she said.

As I have for years with all of my patients, I tried to convince her to try medication for a time. I also asked her to read the testimonies of various patients who had had the surgery, including that of one woman who regretted having had the operation and that of another patient who had developed severe compensatory sweating. But it was no use. Three months later, she had a T2 sympathectomy. After eight months, she wrote me the following note:

> Facial blushing is no longer an issue for me. I have had to
> learn to live with a little more perspiration in the summer,

but I don't care. I have put the problem behind me and I feel more confident now. While the operation has not been 100 percent effective, I am still satisfied and, since my fear of blushing occurs less frequently, I feel much less anxiety. I think I made a good decision, and the good thing is that I was also in good hands, so I thank the entire medical team that treated me from the bottom of my heart.

Regards,
Camila

It will soon be six years since Camila underwent surgery. I contacted her a few days ago. Things have not been easy for her, partly because she still has not been able to fulfill her desire to become a mother. She still thinks, despite suffering from moderate compensatory sweating,[82] that the surgery was a good idea, and she says she is very satisfied with the results.

We should wonder how well these testimonies reflect what typically happens after the surgery. In one study we did some years ago with over one hundred patients who had had an ETS, we found that 99 percent had developed compensatory sweating after the procedure. In 55 percent of the cases the sweating was of moderate intensity, in 32 percent it was slight, and 13 percent had intense sweating. Even so, at about one year after the procedure, 89 percent of these patients reported being "very satisfied" or "quite satisfied" with the results of the operation.[83] These data coincide with the findings of other researchers.[84] The following statements, taken from messages I have received over the years, illustrate this point:

"Absolutely, I believe the operation was worth it."

"But, well, everything has its price, and they warned me about it. I've made a lot of progress in terms of my

---

82 Moderate compensatory sweating means, "I perspire moderately when it is hot, when I exercise, or when I am under psychological stress. Perspiration droplets form and run, but I do not need to change clothes. Although it is uncomfortable, it is not something that embarrasses me." See R. de M. Lyra et al. (2008).
83 See E. Jadresic et al. (2011).
84 See P. B. Licht and H. K. Pilegaard (2008).

personality. I'm blushing 98 percent less. I hope someday they invent another operation to sweat a little less. I'd appreciate it."

"The sweating is *very* uncomfortable, and I'm sometimes very embarrassed about it. I sweat mostly in my armpits, chest, abdomen, back, and thighs. Still, I'll never regret having the operation. It changed my life. I wish these side effects didn't exist, but in the end they don't really matter."

"Hello, Doctor. I do indeed have compensatory sweating now, and according to the rating you sent, I would be at level 3. Still, I should say that in my case it is only in my lower back, and I've never regretted having the surgery."

"I believe that option 3 in the survey is the one that best represents me: moderate compensatory sweating. Sometimes I sweat quite a lot, especially on my abdomen and my back. It's a little embarrassing when it's really hot and my T-shirt gets wet, but I obviously prefer that to turning red because of any little thing, and anyway it doesn't happen all the time."

"My option is number 3, and though I have droplets that run, I'm not at all embarrassed and it hasn't made me sorry I had the operation. In fact, I'm more convinced every day that it was a very good idea to have the operation."

"The blushing disappeared almost entirely after the surgery, and while someone occasionally tells me that I'm blushing, I'm sure that it's not even 10 percent of what it was before. In that respect, I'm totally satisfied. It has completely turned my life around. It would take too long to explain it all. In any case, I want to make it clear that I have no doubt that my current situation is significantly better than before the procedure. It's too bad about this side effect, since otherwise the results would be almost perfect."

"I'm glad you asked me this because a month ago I was about to write to you to ask you what I could do about it. I have sometimes perspired so much that I have to go home and change my clothes, and I can't buy clothes in certain colors (like gray) because the perspiration shows. Even so, I'm not sorry I had the surgery."

"In conclusion, the compensatory sweating is totally tolerable in my case, and I'm happy to have had the operation because I don't have the PB anymore that depressed me so much; now I can live a completely normal life. Thanks, Doc, and rest assured that I'll be happy to answer any other surveys. Hugs, L.S."

Chapter 11
Daniel M.

I read once that seeing is a metaphor for possessing. One might think that this is why doctors, when they look at their patients, are so careful to make them feel that their privacy has not been invaded. That may be true. What I do know is that when I have a blushing patient across from me and I see that he or she is red-faced, I automatically try to give the impression that I do not notice it. It is visceral and instinctive, an attempt to avoid distressing the other person as if by reflex. It is not a matter of avoiding power asymmetry, of seeking to maintain a horizontal doctor-patient relationship; I believe it is an empathetic response from someone who many times suffered the demoralizing humiliation of turning crimson at the slightest provocation.

When I met Daniel in August 2005, I noticed that, despite his thirty-five years, he blushed easily. Maybe that is why, when I looked at him, I tried to ignore the reddening. He did not say anything, but I think he was grateful.[85] A civil engineer, he told me he was married and had a son. He

---

85 An interesting phenomenon to note is that of "mirroring" in interpersonal relationships, particularly in the doctor-patient context, as here. While my patient was blushing and, thus, manifesting his desire to go unnoticed, my striving to ignore what I was seeing could be viewed as the observer—myself—doing the same thing as the observed. Modern neuroscience terms *mirror neurons* a certain type of neurons that are activated both when a certain activity is performed and when another individual is observed performing the same activity. These neurons are presumed to play an important part in capacities such as empathy and imitation, which are crucial to success in relating socially with others. Some authors consider the discovery of mirror neurons as one of the most important scientific findings of recent years. The following fragment of written

worked in a major government ministry and still does today. He had gone to see Dr. Suárez because, contrary to his own and others' predictions, his childhood tendency to blush had never gone away.

It is interesting to note that human behavior depends not only on fear but also on many other attributes, such as will, motivation, and values. Therefore, as I have said, avoidance is not always present in social phobias. In fact, we clinicians frequently see patients who intuitively and repeatedly face social situations in an attempt to overcome their fears. The same is valid for all human phobias, and, in fact, the definition of phobia has been expanded in recent years to include cases in which individuals face feared situations with suffering and anxiety and not only when they avoid them. Some authors have emphasized the fact that, compared to other phobias, social phobias (particularly erythrophobia) are less responsive to exposure therapies (either self-administered or guided by a therapist). This could explain what happened to Daniel and to many other patients, whose fears have persisted despite repeated exposure—for years—to social stimuli.

But let's get back to Daniel:

"I have blushed about anything since I was a kid," he said, breathing more easily now. He was also relieved to have handed over the written note with the preliminary diagnosis that Dr. Suárez usually sends me when referring patients to me.[86] "I didn't have the problem in elementary school," he said. "It started when I went into high school."

---

testimony, which was sent to me a few days ago by a pathological blushing (PB) and facial hyperhidrosis patient, is along the same lines: "I have had to deal with a lot of people in my job. I have had to conduct meetings, but the possibility of suffering these unpleasant symptoms is always latent. My fear of blushing and sweating has led me to stay silent and to try to maintain a low profile. An anecdote I would like to share is that sometimes when I talk to people (especially women), my nose starts to perspire. The other person rarely comments on it, but tends to wipe her own nose with her hand. It's like a mirror reaction, in a way."

86 It is important not to underestimate in clinical practice the significance of the handwritten note, normally from a prescription pad, that the referring doctor gives to the patient. This note is meant for the colleague being consulted and explains the reasons for the referral, and it is a custom that has begun to fall into disuse. It is especially useful for pathological blushing/social anxiety disorder (PB/SAD) patients. Besides being a tangible document, it "speaks" for the patient, which is crucial in dealing with a disorder that the patient finds difficult to acknowledge.

A few days later, he sent me a written testimony reflecting on his high school experiences:

> I would like to go back in time about twenty-five years. I'm in a classroom feeling a certain amount of anxiety after something embarrassing has happened. I see my classmates laughing and hear those around me saying, "Daniel is blushing!" I hear the teacher saying that it happens to everybody and see myself unable to stop the red flooding into my cheeks. That's when I became aware of my blushing, that I began to realize that I couldn't keep from turning red when people were looking at me. It began to cause me more anxiety because it started to affect my life. I would blush in class, on the city bus, at family get-togethers; when I was with a lot of friends, if I had to speak in public, if a girl talked to me (if there were several it was worse still!), when I had to pay a bill and there was a line of people behind me, etc.

As usually happens, it was not long before the consequences of the symptoms became evident in Daniel's life:

> I began to withdraw, to have fewer friends, to avoid social situations, to feign illness if I had to give a presentation in school, and to be always alert to keeping the blushing under control. Sometimes I managed to, to some extent. I also felt better if there was another person around with the same problem. However, the symptom continued to affect how I related to other people. I tried not to stand out even though I had plenty of reasons to, both physically and intellectually. It was the same with my feelings: I was embarrassed to express them because it would make me blush. As a result, I was shy with girls and blushed with my girlfriends (and even more with their parents). I always had short-term relationships in which I never expressed much commitment or affection, even if I had strong feelings.

It was the same at the university. I was always trying to control my blushing right to the end. I even scheduled my thesis defense for a Saturday morning so that fewer people would be there. That's how much the color of embarrassment affected me: it became a serious *problem* and began to take over my life.

In the interview I could see the tremendously negative impact Daniel's symptoms had had on his career. I wrote the following note to Claudio Suárez:

Mr. M. currently feels limited in his job. He has been offered management positions several times in the last four years, but he has always turned them down because of this problem. He says that he isn't prepared for them, even though he feels capable. It is highly probable that he will be offered promotions again in the future, so he has decided to seek medical help once more (ten years ago he went to a psychiatrist in the south of Chile, but the specialist wasn't able to help).

All this was very disheartening for Daniel. He was very discouraged and felt guilty for disappointing his family and denying them the opportunity for greater financial security. As a psychiatrist, in addition to calming his anxiety, I also wanted to keep him from falling into the quagmire of depression, which was likely if he was not treated quickly. I knew that his mother had had various bouts of depression, and I wanted to help him avoid that suffering.

The repercussions of his symptoms touched every aspect of his life:

My wife and I got married in a very small private civil ceremony; I didn't want a church wedding for the same reason as always: blushing. I had no trouble being with my children [he had two more after I met him]; at home I could pretend that nothing was wrong, or maybe, in a

way, I was able to control myself more. Still, I never went
to school meetings, year-end activities, programs, etc.

With the new perspective given by the passage of time and being
symptom-free, our patient could let go of the embarrassment and share
with others the silent world in which he was submerged. He left the neurotic
egocentricity, so to speak, in which the disorder frequently envelops the
sufferer and was capable of seeing beyond the immediacy of the symptoms:

> I imagine that this touches a nerve for many people
> reading this. They may understand the anxiety I came to
> feel, the helplessness of needing to hang back for fear of
> blushing, of not being able to be the protagonist in my
> own life.

Eager to let us know the outcome of his story, he continued:

> The years went by until finally the Internet arrived and I
> discovered that now, in the twenty-first century, there is a
> surgical treatment for this problem. I immediately made
> up my mind to go see a doctor. He referred me to Dr.
> Jadresic, who recommended that I try drug therapy until
> I came to a decision and asked me to share my experience
> afterward.

After interviewing Daniel, I wrote a medical report stating that he
was suffering from pathological blushing (PB) and axillary and inguinal
hyperhidrosis, and that a sympathectomy was a suitable option for him.
However, I did indeed suggest that he try taking fifty milligrams of sertraline
per day on a permanent basis. At the same time, I prescribed twenty
milligrams of propranolol and half a fifty-milligram alprazolam tablet (to
be taken simultaneously) before particularly stressful social situations.

I saw Daniel only that one time, but I am convinced that our meeting
was fruitful. What he told me in an e-mail two years later is evidence
enough:

95

The fact of the matter, and I've been lucky, is that the medication took effect quickly. After a few weeks I began to notice that I didn't blush so deeply, I didn't become anxious, and I no longer avoided social situations as much. It got better and better as time went by. I felt more confident and began to speak in public without any difficulty. *I was thrilled!* And although it might sound like an exaggeration, I was starting out on a whole new life, one without blushing. I felt so good that I accepted a long-postponed management position. [Daniel was promoted to a managerial position with nationwide responsibility.] I started to teach, and I'm no longer afraid of the public or of standing in lines … or of drawing attention to myself.

Daniel accepts the cost of having to take medication on a daily basis. Given the benefits he has reaped, he does not mind. He tells us clearly what he currently thinks:

I've been taking medication every day for nine years now without feeling a dependency. If my opinion matters and can help other people, I fully recommend this solution. The likelihood of my having the surgery has dropped to the point that I'm almost not considering it, but I haven't completely closed the door on the possibility.

After so many years of taking a fifty-milligram tablet of sertraline every day (to which, every now and then, he adds the combination of propranolol and alprazolam prior to taking part in very anxiety-provoking social situations), Daniel evaluated his degree of satisfaction with the drug therapy as follows: degree of overall satisfaction, "quite helpful"; impact on job performance, "quite helpful"; impact on his sentimental relationship, "somewhat helpful"; and impact on other social relationships (primarily friendships), "quite helpful." The method used was that applied in chapter 6. In addition, he was asked to write an answer to the question, "If you feel that drug therapy for blushing has been helpful, specifically how do you feel it has provided relief?" Three possible answers were provided: 1 = the treatment has helped because I blush less intensely and/or less frequently; 2 = I still blush but I do not mind so much now; and 3 = I blush less intensely and/or less frequently and, besides, I do not mind so much now. Daniel unhesitatingly responded that, in his opinion, the medication had enabled him to blush less intensely and/or less frequently (answer 1).

Chapter 12
Francesca C.

Francesca (her real name) said that blushing was an illness that cast a shadow over her life. For many years, she believed that she was the only one who experienced something so extreme, so she was moved to tears when she read other patients' stories and realized that she was not the only one trapped by blushing. She became even more excited when she learned that it is a treatable condition.

She came to see me along with her maternal grandmother. Despite the fact that Francesca's mother had been the one to buy her the first edition of *When Blushing Hurts*, neither parent took their daughter's suffering very seriously. Two weeks after our first meeting, Francesca summarized her symptoms in writing:

> I'm a twenty-year-old girl in my second year of studying to be a physical therapist. I'm quiet and introverted, and I blush at everything. And it's not an exaggeration when I say at everything. I had a hard time in school because of blushing. Whenever I had to give a presentation to the class, I would get very nervous and begin to turn red as soon as I started to speak. I would realize it immediately and the suffering would begin. The only thing I could think during those times was how ridiculous I looked and that everyone would laugh at me. I would also blush, and still do, when I would run into someone in a public place, when I talked on the phone, when I greeted someone, etc.

I don't like to go out much because of it, not even to do a little shopping, but sometimes I do just because I think that maybe that way I can get over this social phobia I have because of blushing so much. It's been five years and I think it's gotten even worse. I'm at the university now, where I always have to make presentations or argue different points of view, which is always very difficult for me.

Next, she told me about when she had told her parents about her symptoms and her optimism at her imminent treatment:

When I told my parents about all this, they didn't consider it to be significant, especially my father. He thinks it's just a lack of personality, some little thing that I'll get over in time. The only one who understands how serious of a problem the blushing is, and I'm very grateful to her for it, is my grandmother, who told me she'd be happy to give me whatever help I need. So I got an appointment with Dr. Jadresic on April 13, 2011, and I'll never forget it. I told him about all this. Looking at him, I could tell that he completely understood and, though I felt that I was blushing, this time it was with someone who knew what I was feeling. I'm very grateful to him for being so empathetic. Now we'll see if the treatment works. I'm very happy to think that this will all be over soon and I will have a normal life. I have a lot of faith, and I know this will work.

As I summarize Francesca's story, I cannot forget the teachings of Dr. Sergio Peña y Lillo,[87] who stated categorically that anxiety must always be treated when it appears as clinical anxiety; that is, as a symptom, as a complaint, and the reason for seeking medical help. He argued that the primary goal of medicine is not for the patient to understand himself or

---

87 A renowned Chilean psychiatrist who died in 2012. See S. Peña y Lillo (1981).

herself or to solve conflicts that impede or hinder personal development and growth, but rather to restore health and well-being by eliminating symptoms and, whenever possible, curing the illness.

Francesca had become progressively more withdrawn over time. She had not had any boyfriends and had almost no relationships beyond her immediate family. Believing that endoscopic thoracic sympathectomy (ETS) was the most effective treatment for abnormal blushing, her focus was on the surgery, but she accepted my suggestion that she take fifty milligrams of sertraline per day on an ongoing basis, plus a combination of alprazolam and propranolol before going into social situations that she found particularly threatening.

Some time later, as we had agreed, she sent me a second personal testimony:

> Three months after beginning the drug therapy, the changes have been spectacular. I now find that I can easily do the things that used to hold me back. The blushing comes less frequently than before, and it seems like it doesn't last as long. My life has turned completely around. Now I can talk for a long time without my face turning red because of just any little thing. I feel capable of doing many things, like going out alone, asking questions, or talking on the telephone in front of other people; before, I couldn't do these things without fear of blushing. The changes have really been wonderful, and the personality I had hidden away is beginning to come out, little by little, but with assurance and confidence.

She then commented specifically on the drug treatment:

> The "magic potion" (alprazolam + propranolol)—ha ha, that's what I call it because it truly is magic—I've only used it twice since the sertraline alone is enough for me to live a normal life. I used the "potion" once when I had to make a presentation at the university, and I did a really good job. I used it again when I went to a discotheque for

the first time with my cousin, and I had a lot of fun. That's what I can tell you for now. I hope to continue progressing with this. I'm very grateful for having found help with the blushing. I'm grateful to my grandmother, of course, and also to you, Dr. Jadresic, for having written the book that awoke me from my nightmare.

I am reluctant to quote my patients' gratitude in order not to seem self-congratulatory, but I have included this quote here to highlight an idea: that reading a book can be the beginning of help or healing. I have frequently been told by my blushing patients that even something as simple as buying a book in a bookstore is in some way out of reach for them. Various patients have confided to me that they had wanted to buy *When Blushing Hurts* but that they had not dared to because they were afraid they would blush in front of the sales clerk. Of course, the availability of digital books on the Internet has radically changed this situation in recent years.

It has been almost three years since Francesca came to see me, but she recently sent me an e-mail telling me about her progress. She said, "I'm doing great compared to before the treatment. To anyone who suffers from this, I would tell them to gather up their courage and see a doctor!" She told me that she was still taking fifty milligrams of sertraline per day, so I asked if she would answer a survey evaluating her degree of satisfaction with the medication. On a scale of 1 to 5, in order of increasing satisfaction, the response that best reflected her case was "very helpful/very satisfied." Later, she was pleased to hear that I was working on an updated version of *When Blushing Hurts*. She was happy to have aspects of her case recounted in the book, and she wanted her real name to be used. I commended her for her openness, which takes real courage.

Since Francesca came to see me after reading about blushing, which had given her the opportunity to identify with other patients' stories and to decide to seek help, I would like to emphasize the importance of the fact that these patients seek professional help specifically for their blushing and not for another problem. This may seem obvious, but it is not. I frequently hear people complain that their symptoms were not explicitly addressed in previous professional treatments. Statements such as, "The doctor went back to my childhood" or "They didn't consider my blushing important and focused on my personality" are fairly common. It is crucial that the professional be informed and know what to ask. One patient explained how hearing the right words from his doctor affected their relationship: "It's like a light came on, and I trusted her implicitly when, because of her insightful questions, I knew that she understood my problem."

Another important consideration of Francesca's story is that, while she is a good example of what happens with many patients who respond well to medication, her case is not particularly dramatic. In fact, her case is much less severe than others I have seen in recent years.

The following quotes contrast her case with others that I have seen over the years that are either more severe or unique:

> Besides blushing, which was not due to embarrassment but rather was the source of my embarrassment, I also had other symptoms like excessive sweating and really unpleasant trembling in my hands and throughout my body in general. My classmates were aware of these symptoms and, not realizing how much it bothered me, they made jokes about it, which I reacted to with a forced laugh. It all gave me a feeling of tremendous helplessness and anger, and it seriously affected my self-esteem, but most of all it was extremely limiting. I was interested in my classes and I felt it was important to participate and give my opinion, but I knew that if I raised my hand to say something I would blush, and so I wouldn't take part.
>
> The anxiety and anguish from blushing got to be so bad that several times I stayed home from school just because I knew I would be exposed to a difficult situation or I had to make a speech. A clear example of this is that once they had a *graded* spelling test, and the student who had the most words right would be in a contest that would be held in front of all the seventh- and eighth-graders. On the one hand, it was relatively easy for me to write the words since I have good spelling, but on the other I didn't want to get them all right, even though it was for a grade, in order not to be exposed to blushing. Finally,

though it was difficult for me to do it, I spelled some of the words wrong on purpose, even though I knew how to spell all of them.

Besides, all the stress caused by constantly having to be alert to blushing situations brought down my grades, and I didn't have the energy and joy that I had had before.

—A fourteen-year-old patient

I didn't blush much as a teenager and it didn't use to bother me too much except for right at the moment, when I didn't want anyone to notice what was happening. Back then I felt that when I blushed I lost my focus, my mind would go foggy, and I couldn't control what I now know is uncontrollable.

As the years went by, I was frequently embarrassed with my mother-in-law's family when they told off-color jokes at family lunches. I would turn red because I knew I would, not because I was disturbed by the sexual connotation of the jokes, but because I knew I was going to look ridiculous. I had to leave teaching for obvious reasons and I took other jobs, always suffering, always stressed, always red and perspiring.

In about 1980 I decided to seek psychiatric help. If memory serves me right, I have seen about seven psychiatrists, and they all treated me for depression. Some antidepressants helped by decreasing my anxiety, but the blushing I hated was always there, sometimes less frequent but sometimes the same as before. I've tried psychotherapy and I've thought about trying acupuncture, hypnosis, yoga, herbs, positive thinking, even just not paying attention to it, but it's taken over my life.

One day I did an Internet search on *facial blushing* and found Dr. Suárez, who performs a surgery that has been a solution in many cases. That's when I realized that PB, which was always considered just a symptom in my case, was actually the crux of my problem, and I decided to see him. I'm undecided as to which option to take, the operation or drug therapy, but I do know that I want to do something to help myself. Hiding, avoiding, running away, evading, being alert, wearing myself out, and suffering; these are all verbs that I am intimately familiar with. As I told my doctor, "I'm going to die without knowing what it is to be relaxed, without being able to enjoy my relationships and friendships, without knowing how to live." When I met these doctors, I found out that I'm not the only one. I think that the best thing you can do if you suffer from this disorder is to look for a solution, and the sooner you do, the sooner you will be able to enjoy life. I'm grateful to Drs. Jadresic and Suárez for giving me a chance that I didn't know I had.

—A seventy-year-old patient

In what follows, I quote other experiences recounted to me by patients over the course of several years. Their stories vividly illustrate the many personal implications reddening can have on blushers' lives.

Blamed Unjustly for Misdeeds

"Since I was the only one in the class that blushed, they always blamed me."

"Once when I was in the supermarket with my husband, we ran into someone from my work and I turned red. My husband started to imagine all kinds of things. He thought I had something going on with this colleague and it started a huge problem between us."

Solidarity Blushing

"When I was young I had "mirror blushing." If someone turned red, I did too. I might even blush for a classmate who was in trouble even if he didn't at all."

"Once a lady fainted and I blushed for her."

Worried about the Wedding

"I'm not even dating and I'm already worried about walking into the church with people looking at me when I get married."

"I went to see hundreds of churches and finally chose the one that had the shortest distance between the church and the entrance so that I would be at less risk [of blushing]."

"I thank God that I married a Muslim. That way I didn't have to get married in the church."

The Brave One

"I expose myself [to blushing] on purpose. That's why I went to work for a TV station."

Academics and Professional Life

"I preferred getting bad grades in school to giving a speech."

"I quit school and got a high school equivalency diploma instead."

"I was accepted to study architecture, but I didn't because of the blushing."

"I left the university."

"I became a technician instead so I wouldn't have to interact with people."

"They offered me a management position but I didn't take it, saying I wasn't qualified."

"I quit the job because I was going to have to give talks."

Social Life

"I turned down an invitation to England because there was a boy where I was going and I was afraid I would blush."

"I only go out at night; at night, all cats are black."

"I put on makeup before I go out. First I use white makeup for mimes and then put regular makeup base on top."

"I go out and get sunburned to avoid turning red in front of people."

"I pinch my cheeks so that they turn red before I blush. That way it's not noticeable."

"I ask first so that I don't get asked questions. That way I'm not taken by surprise." [PB occurs most frequently in unforeseen situations.]

"I greet people first before they can greet me."

"At social gatherings, my first cocktail always goes faster than everyone else's."

"Extreme" Cases

"My family thought that I was so withdrawn because the priests had abused me."

"When I was young I thought that PB was hereditary, so I didn't want to have children."

"I would stab myself with needles."

"For a while I gave myself electric shocks."

"I would take up to twenty or thirty zopiclones[88] a day when I had to be in social situations."

"Once when I had to give a speech I didn't blush, but my legs turned bright red."

"Once I saw someone I knew in the street. I turned and ran because of the PB and almost got hit by a bus."

"Once I blushed with the father of one of my child's classmates because he looked like a guy I liked."

"I turn red when they take my picture for my ID card."

"I don't wear a bikini because I'm afraid I'll blush if I get whistled at."

"They knew about my problem at school, so they let me give my presentations with my back to the class!"

"They offered to have a pastor do an exorcism to solve my problem."

"I'm uncomfortable with it because I export tomatoes."

---

88 Zopiclone is a nonbenzodiazepine used to treat insomnia.

Chapter 13
Nicholas R.

Nicholas was thirty years old and was working for an insurance company when he came to see me. He had been divorced for quite some time and had two small children who still—four years later—lived with their mother. He told me that he had blushed easily since his school days, especially when attention was focused on him, if he unexpectedly ran into an acquaintance, or if he had to speak to a group of colleagues at work.

I asked him, "Why are you just now seeking medical help?"

"I don't want to keep on living like this!" he said. He explained that he was tired of living his life constantly anticipating humiliation because of the blushing.

He added that he was very lonely and felt like a failure for not having found a new partner. He felt rejected because every time he tried to start a conversation with a woman he would blush. He was afraid that it made him unattractive because it made him seem weaker and, therefore, less masculine.

"And giving the impression that I'm weak and insecure means that I have less confidence, so I become even more insecure."

He reported feeling trapped by having to live in a constant state of hypervigilance: "I feel this way 80 percent of the day. The only time I don't is when I'm alone or with someone who's really close."

Although they may seem to be, people who seek medical help for blushing are not particularly narcissistic; they are focused on themselves because the visibility of their physical symptoms makes them feel in danger, vulnerable. Consequently, they go through life always on high alert.

Nicholas said that he would first like to try treatment with medication because he wanted to improve quickly and surgery seemed like an extreme step to take.

I prescribed ten milligrams per day of escitalopram, and we agreed to meet again in three months. Naturally, I told him he could contact me at any time by e-mail, and, in fact, we agreed that we would have a "checkup" by e-mail in six weeks. In the end, it turned out not to be necessary.

After three months, he said he was significantly better and felt that his autonomic nervous system had calmed down. He said, "I no longer have that internal terrorist inside who used to go with me everywhere" (referring to the physical symptoms of blushing, accelerated heart rate, perspiration, and shaking that had distracted him daily, prevented him from keeping his train of thought, and made it difficult to have relationships with other people).

He started on a positive spiral, now that he had the courage to participate in all aspects of life. He also offered his opinion more at work, something that several people commented on, pleasantly surprised. All this meant that, after a few months, he began to receive and issue invitations and to feel more integrated in activities, which infused him with increased self-confidence. Despite this improvement, a year later he noted that his initial enthusiasm of the first months, which was possibly due to the contrast with his previous situation, had dwindled and been replaced by a feeling of apathy or indifference. He felt that things were less likely to appeal to him and that his prevailing mood now tended to be disinterest. It was true that the constant anxiety had lessened considerably; in other words, he suffered less, but he also had the impression that he enjoyed things less as well. This lack of interest, which is sometimes associated with the use of selective serotonin reuptake inhibitors (SSRIs), is similar to what doctors call *frontal lobe syndrome* and can be unpleasant to experience. It depends on the dosage and goes away when the medication is no longer taken. Besides, Nicholas continued to be frustrated by his lack of a romantic attachment, something he blamed himself for, although to a lesser degree than before.

I suggested cutting the escitalopram dose in half in order to improve his enthusiasm and complementing the medication with psychotherapy. He would meet a number of times with a psychologist who would start with task concentration training (TCT) exercises, followed by various sessions of cognitive behavioral therapy (CBT). Nicholas agreed and, while he didn't mind taking the escitalopram tablet every day, he was pleased when I suggested that, if he worked hard in the psychotherapy, he might eventually be able to stop taking the medication.

He attended eight weekly sessions of TCT and then six weekly sessions of CBT (some were group sessions). He was also asked to keep a daily record of the exercises he did on his own.

Among the group exercises were, for example, having to be observed silently by the others for fifteen minutes while he looked at everyone in the eyes in order to face his fear of being the center of attention, or speaking spontaneously in front of the group on a topic assigned at random. Homework exercises included simulating anxiety to test the validity of his belief that, "if I show that I'm anxious, they'll think I'm stupid because I'm showing my weakness," and talking to strangers in lines, at a subway station, or in an elevator.

These exposure exercises are obviously not easy, and a certain amount of anxiety is to be expected, but the fact that they are done gradually and at a pace that is tolerable to each patient makes them bearable. They have three enormous advantages: First, directly experiencing confrontation demonstrates the erroneous nature of many of the patients' beliefs and expectations. Second, even if the beliefs about a situation do turn out to be true, exposure to the situation enables patients to handle their anxiety better. Finally, exposure is an ideal opportunity to put social skills into practice.

Nicholas benefited from all of this, and he gradually learned to be more relaxed and serene in how he related to the world around him. He continued taking escitalopram for another year, but then he gradually stopped taking it as I instructed him by e-mail.

At the psychologist's request, he signed up in 2012 and 2013, once each year, to take part in an activity in which he deliberately came into contact with other people. So he took a course in public speaking some time ago and, more recently, he worked up the courage to participate in a dancing workshop near his home. I contacted him a few days ago, and he immediately sent the following reply:

Santiago

March 18, 2014

Hello, Doc,

I would like to thank you and tell you that my life has changed 100 percent for the better. I rarely blush now and I can control situations better. I'm very happy with the results. I no longer feel like a prisoner in my body and it's very pleasant to live this way. I've also been in a relationship for six months, and I have a different outlook on the future now. I am deeply grateful for your work and effort. It really changed my life, and it would never have happened without you and the psychologist.

Nicholas

Afterword (2007)

Blushing seems to be a bodily condition rather than a virtue.

−Aristotle

To paraphrase Aristotle, who held that blushing is more of a physical affliction than a moral virtue, I hope that I have been able to show that blushing can become a symptom and a source of suffering. Despite its being an enigmatic, unique personal expression that is, at the same time, universal,[89] it is rarely studied. For many readers, including health professionals, the content of these pages must have been, in a sense, a discovery, but not for the reader who was already interested in the topic. The latter will have noticed the disparity between the proliferation in cyberspace of personal testimonies on sympathectomies and the scarcity of information for patients from reliable medical sources.

The information available is generally displayed on the websites of surgical teams who perform sympathectomies or on Internet discussion forums, usually promoted by patients who have been dissatisfied with

---

89 During the nineteenth century, scientists, philosophers, and theologians hotly debated whether or not the nonwhite population blushed. Some theologians held that the fact that only whites blushed placed them in a unique and fundamentally different moral position over other races or animals. The discussion had not only moral but also political connotations. If nonwhites did not blush, they were not completely human; thus it was legitimate to enslave them and colonize their lands. Darwin made it clear that blacks and other dark-skinned people also experience increased blood flow to the face in social situations that produce visible blushing in whites. The difference stems from the fact that, for the former, this blood flow results only in darker skin or is simply not visible. Therefore, some authors have recommended using a more general term for the phenomenon, suggesting *social facial vasodilatation*. See M. R. Leary et al. (1992).

the surgery. There is clearly a need for other health-care professionals to become involved. I know that my work as a psychiatrist in this area is, incidentally, among those pioneering in the field; this is an additional reason for presenting the biographical fragments and thoughts on the topic that I have included in the book. Through my own experience and what I have learned from the experiences of others, I believe that medicine has an enormous potential for transforming this area.

I had originally planned to include the testimonies of many other patients whose enthusiasm and willingness to cooperate is commendable. When I delved into their personal narratives, their stories became a magical fabric interweaving affection, catharsis, and solidarity. I had also intended to include other material touching on what Darwin and Twain coincided in describing as "the most human of expressions," but I have omitted them for the sake of conciseness. Still, I have attempted to illustrate, with subtlety, how blushing is not a simple matter for some people, and how it can develop into a symptom that deserves our attention and sometimes warrants treatment, in some cases even surgery. I have also, albeit indirectly, tried to show that we would do well to eliminate the stigma associated with blushing so that people can do so without distress.

One brief personal comment: This book unexpectedly began to come about some time after my surgery when, on the one hand, I felt that I had a lot to say and, on the other, I noticed that I had to get used to living with dry hands, a common side effect of endoscopic thoracic sympathectomy (ETS). As a result, I traded my paintbrush—I had recently taken up painting—for the computer keyboard. My interest in the simultaneity of imagery had become transformed into an attraction for the flow of narrative.

Whether or not the muses have succeeded in whispering in my ear, I have enjoyed immersing myself in the creative mood necessary for writing about one's own experiences. I am grateful that this book has been such a pleasant experience in communication. Somewhere, beyond all the theoretical concepts presented, I hope to have touched the reader in some measure. If not, I am consoled by some anonymous words that I have now made my own: "I believe in texts that dare to speak, even if they do not achieve all that they set out to do."

Postscript (2014)

I have been practicing psychiatry for over thirty years, and I have been seeing patients with excessive facial blushing for more than ten. As I look back over this time, I am struck by this paradox: despite the fact that we live in a more individualistic society, one in which the opinion of others seems to carry less weight, blushing continues to cause great discomfiture to the person turning red.

Some will insist that blushing is normal. They will say that it is an adaptive mechanism in social situations both for the individual (to facilitate acceptance) and for the group (by facilitating social cohesion). Following this logic, they will argue that it does not make sense to treat people for blushing. While I do not deny that turning red may have positive aspects, I would like to point out that the experience of blushing is not the same for everyone and that those who seek medical help do so because the experience of repeated blushing has undermined their quality of life. Otherwise, these patients would not be willing to run the risks involved in the sympathectomy or be willing to put up with compensatory sweating in order to control the blushing that they find so disturbing. Only someone who has been genuinely and severely affected by a condition is ready to undergo surgery. In other words, we cannot sidestep the fact that some people suffer from a type of blushing that, quite literally, hurts.

In addition, the fact that a symptom is adaptive does not place it beyond the reach of medical treatment. Quite the contrary: We physicians treat numerous symptoms that cause immediate discomfort to the individual—pain and vomiting are good examples—which may be considered to be adaptive and, as such, part of the solution rather than the problem. Thus, the pain of a leg fracture leads us to immobilize the extremity, which contributes to healing and helps prevent greater injury. Nonetheless, no one would doubt the legitimacy of treating pain in these cases. I believe that the same is true for blushing. Recognizing its potential adaptive value does not mean that it should not be treated.

I am aware that medicalization focuses the source of the problem on the individual rather than on the social environment and thus gives priority to individual medical treatment over more collective or societal solutions. I do wish that our societies were more tolerant and sensitive to the emotions of others; in that world, blushing would not be a problem to those who suffer from it. But until that happens, until we have a society that is more respectful and less aggressive, with less bullying and less concerned with appearances—one in which blushing is not a source of embarrassment—people will continue to seek out psychological and medical support.

As a medical student, I learned that, rather than having illnesses, we have ill people. From this standpoint, the discussion of whether a certain type of blushing should be considered a separate morbid condition or should be kept as a component of social anxiety disorder (SAD) becomes less relevant. Priority should always be given to curing the patient or, alternatively, alleviating the symptoms; if neither is possible, the least we can do is let the sufferer know that he or she is not alone. That said, in an attempt to understand those who struggle with blushing, I believe it is pertinent to ask the following questions: Do people blush abnormally because they have SAD? Or do they develop SAD and its avoidance behaviors because of their marked tendency to blush easily and excessively?

From experience, I am inclined to believe that certain people have a particular biological predisposition, under the influence of their genes, that causes them to blush more when faced with certain stimuli, and especially after negative learning experiences, they develop a SAD. In support of this hypothesis, it is worth noting that, unlike what was previously believed, we now know that those who seek medical help for blushing tend to blush more easily than others. Also, I cannot ignore the fact that clinical histories and the chronological progression of many of my patients' symptoms suggest that sufferers can develop SAD as a negative adaptive response to frequent experiences of blushing. This hypothesis correlates with other authors' proposals to consider a form of SAD as secondary to facial blushing.

This idea in no way denies the importance of personality and of each individual's cognitive makeup. There are certainly many people who blush intensely but are not disturbed by it, while others redden to a lesser degree and yet find themselves inhibited both emotionally and socially. Undoubtedly, blushing is a tremendously negative experience for many people, but the negative or positive connotations associated with blushing also depend, as we have previously seen, on the psychological importance we place on it. I am hopeful that psychotherapies used to correct patients' distorted interpretations of blushing will be perfected in the coming years, and that the psychological treatments already available will become more accessible. I also hope that this book will prompt further medical research in order to help the many people whose lives have been taken over, painfully and for many long years, by facial blushing.

Bibliography

Adair A., George M.L., Camprodon R., Broadfield J.A., Rennie J.A. (2005). Endoscopic sympathectomy in the treatment of facial blushing. *Annals of the Royal College of Surgeons of England* 87: 358–60.

American Psychiatric Association (2013). *Diagnostic and Statistical Manual for Mental Disorders, 5ᵗʰ edition*. Washington, DC: APA.

Amies P.L., Gelder M.G., Shaw P.M. (1983). Social phobia: A comparative clinical study. *British Journal of Psychiatry* 142: 174–9.

Bloch S. (2005). The Art of Psychiatry. *World Psychiatry* 4(3): 130–4.

Boeringa J.A. (1983). Blushing: A modified behavioral intervention using paradoxical intention. *Psychotherapy: Theory, Research and Practice* 20: 441–4.

Bögels S.M., Mulkens S., de Jong P.J. (1997) Task concentration training and fear of blushing: practitioner report. *Clinical Psychology and Psychotherapy* 4: 251–8.

Bögels S.M., Voncken M. (2008). Social skills training versus cognitive therapy for social anxiety disorder characterized by fear of blushing, trembling, or sweating. *International Journal of Cognitive Therapy* 1: 138–50.

Burlan A.D., Mailis A., Papagapiou M. (2000). Are we paying a high price for surgical sympathectomy? A systematic literature review of late complications. *The Journal of Pain: Official Journal of the American Pain Society* 1: 245–57.

Cía A.H. (2004). *Trastorno de Ansiedad Social. Manual Diagnóstico Terapéutico y de Autoayuda.* Buenos Aires: Editorial Polemos.

Connor K.M., Davidson J.R.T., Churchill L., Sherwood A., Foa E., Weisler R. (2000). Psychometric properties of the Social Phobia Inventory (SPIN). New self-rating scale. *British Journal of Psychiatry* 176: 379–86.

Connor K.M., Davidson J.R.T., Chung H., Yang R., Clary C. (2006). Multidimensional effects of sertraline in social anxiety disorder. *Depression and Anxiety* 23: 6–10.

Conrad P. (2007). *The Medicalization of Society.* Baltimore: The Johns Hopkins University Press.

Crozier W.R. (2006). *Blushing and the Social Emotions: The Self Unmasked.* Houndmills, Basingstoke, Hampshire: Palgrave Macmillan.

Crozier W.R., de Jong P.J. (2013). *The Psychological Significance of the Blush.* Cambridge: Cambridge University Press.

Davidson J.R.T., Miner C.M., De Veaugh-Geiss J., Tupler L.A., Colket J.T., Potts N.L. (1997). The Brief Social Phobia Scale: A psychometric evaluation. *Psychological Medicine* 27: 161–6.

Darwin C. (1872/1955). *The Expression of the Emotions in Man and Animals.* New York: The Philosophical Library.

de Jong P.J. (1999). Communicative and remedial effects of social blushing. *Journal of Nonverbal Behaviour* 23: 197–217.

Drott C., Claes G., Rex L. (2002). Facial blushing treated by sympathetic denervation: long lasting benefits in 831 patients. *Journal of Cosmetic Dermatology* 1: 115–9.

Drummond P.D. (2001). The effect of true and false feedback on blushing in women. *Personality and Individual Differences* 30(8): 1329–43.

Drummond P.D., Lance J. W. (1987). Facial flushing and sweating mediated by the sympathetic nervous system. *Brain* 110(3): 793–803.

Drummond P.D., Back K., Harrison J., Dogg Helgadottir F., Lange B., Lee C., Leavy K., Novatscou C. et al. (2007). Blushing during social interaction in people with a fear of blushing. *Behaviour Research and Therapy* 45: 1601–8.

Drummond P.D., Minosora K., Little G., Keay W. (2013). Topical ibuprofen inhibits blushing during embarrassment and facial blushing during aerobic exercise in people with fear of blushing. *European Neuropsychopharmacology* 23(12): 1747–53.

Edelmann R.J. (1990/2004). *Coping with Blushing*. London: Sheldon Press.

Jadresic E., Súarez C., Palacios E., Palacios F., Matus P (2011). Evaluating the efficacy of endoscopic thoracic sympathectomy for generalized social anxiety disorder with blushing complaints: a comparison with sertraline and no treatment. Santiago, Chile 2003–2009. *Innovations in Clinical Neuroscience* 8(11): 24–35.

Jeganathan R., Jordan S., Jones M., Grant S., Diamond O., McManus K., Graham A., McGuigan J. (2008). Bilateral thoracoscopic sympathectomy: results and long-term follow-up. *Interactive Cardiovascular and Thoracic Surgery* 7(1): 67–70.

Keltner D. (2003). Expression and the course of life. Studies of emotion, personality and psychopathology from a social-functional perspective. In *Emotions Inside Out. 130 Years after Darwin's The Expression of the*

Emotions in Man and Animals. P. Ekman, J.J. Campos, R.J. Davidson, B.M. de Waal Fran (Eds.). New York: The New York Academy of Sciences.

Leary M.R., Cutlip W.D. II, Brito T.W., Templeton J.L. (1992). Social blushing. *Psychological Bulletin* 3: 446–60.

Licht P.B., Ladegaard L., Pilegaard H.K. (2006). Thoracoscopic sympathectomy for isolated facial blushing. *The Annals of Thoracic Surgery* 81: 1863–6.

Licht P.B, Pilegaard H.K. (2008). Management of facial blushing. *Thoracic Surgery Clinics* 18(22): 223–8.

Liebowitz M.R. (1987). Social phobia. *Modern Problems of Pharmacopsychiatry* 22: 141–73.

Liebowitz M.R., Salman E., Nicolini H., Rosenthal N., Hanover R., Monti L. (2014). Effect of an acute intranasal aerosol dose of PH94B on social and performance anxiety in women with social anxiety disorder. *American Journal of Psychiatry* 171(6): 675–82.

Lyra R. de M., Campos J.R., Kang D.W. et al. (2008). Guidelines for the prevention, diagnosis and treatment of compensatory hyperhidrosis. Sociedade Brasileira de Cirurgia Torácica. *Jornal Brasileiro de Pneumologia* 34(11): 967–977.

Mellander S., Andersson P.O., Afzelius L.E., Hellstrand P. (1982). Neural beta-adrenergic dilatation of the facial vein in man. *Acta Physiologica Scandinavica* 114: 393–9.

NICE, National Institute for Health and Care Excellence (2014). Endoscopic thoracic sympathectomy for primary facial blushing. Issued: February 2014. NICE interventional procedure guidance 480. Retrieved from www.guidance.nice.org.uk/ipg480.

Nicolau M. (2006). Blushing: an embarrassing condition, but treatable. *The Lancet* 367: 1297–8.

Ojimba T.A., Cameron A.E. (2004). Drawbacks of endoscopic thoracic sympathectomy. *The British Journal of Surgery* 91: 264–9.

Pande A.C., Feltner D.E., Jefferson J.W., Davidson J.R., Pollack M., Stein M.B., Lydiard R.B., Futterer R., Robinson P., Slomkowski M., DuBoff E., Phelps M., Janney C.A., Werth J.L. (2004). Efficacy of the novel anxiolytic pregabalin in social anxiety disorder: a placebo-controlled, multicenter study. *Journal of Clinical Psychopharmacology* 24(2): 141–9.

Pelissolo A., Moukheiber A. (2013). Open-label treatment with citalopram in patients with social anxiety disorder and fear of blushing. *Journal of Clinical Psychopharmacology* 33(5): 695–8.

Peña y Lillo S. (1981). *La Angustia. Antropología y Clínica*. Santiago: Editorial Universitaria.

Piet J., Hougaard E., Hecksher M.S., Rosenberg N.K. (2010). A randomized pilot study of mindfulness-based cognitive therapy and group cognitive-behavioral therapy for young adults with social phobia. *Scandinavian Journal of Psychology* 51: 403–10.

Pohjavaara P., Telaranta T., Väisänen E. (2003). The role of the sympathetic nervous system in anxiety. Is it possible to relieve anxiety with endoscopic sympathetic block? *Nordic Journal of Psychiatry* 57(1): 55–60.

Pohjavaara P., Telaranta T. (2005). Endoscopic sympathetic block as treatment of social phobia. *European Surgery* 37(3): 137–42.

Ray D., Williams G. (1993). Pathophysiological causes and clinical significance of flushing. *British Journal of Hospital Medicine* 50: 504–98.

Sacks O. (1987). *Awakenings*. New York: Simon & Schuster.

Sanjuan J. (2000). *Evolución cerebral y psicopatología*. Madrid: Editorial Triacastela.

Schick C.H., Horbach T. (2003). Sequelae of endoscopic sympathetic block. *Clinical Autonomic Research: Official Journal of the Clinical Autonomic Research Society* 13(suppl. 1): 136–9.

Smidfelt K., Drott C. (2011). Late results of endoscopic thoracic sympathectomy for hyperhidrosis and facial blushing. *British Journal of Surgery* 98(12): 1719–24.

Stein D.J., Bouwer C. (1997). Blushing and social phobia: a neuroethological speculation. *Medical Hypotheses* 49: 101–8

Suárez C., Suárez F., Pérez L., Lemus J. (2005). Resultado en 100 simpatectomías videotoracoscópicas (SVT) para el tratamiento de la hiperhidrosis de miembros superiores (HHMS). *Revista Chilena de Cirugía* 57: 199–202.

van der Meer C. (1985). Pharmacotherapy of "idiopathic" excessive blushing and hyperhidrosis. *Acta Neurochirurgica* (Vienna) 74(3–4): 151–2.

Wittmoser R. (1985). Treatment of sweating and blushing by endoscopic surgery. *Acta Neurochirurgica* (Vienna) 74: 153–4.

World Health Organization (1993). *The ICD-10 Classification of Mental and Behavioural Disorders: Clinical Descriptions and Diagnostic Guidelines*. Geneva: WHO.

Yalom I.D. (2005). *Schopenhauer's Cure*. New York: HarperCollins.

Appendix

The following two figures show the opinions of 199 consecutive pathological blushing patients, with or without hyperhidrosis, who sought medical help for this condition. All patients met DSM-IV criteria for social anxiety disorder (SAD) as defined by the American Psychiatric Association. The assessments were carried out at a mean of eleven months (range 1–64) after endoscopic thoracic sympathectomy (ETS) or initiation of sertraline. See E. Jadresic et al. (2011).

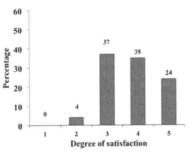

1 = I regret having had sertraline treatment
2 = It was not helpful at all
3 = It was somewhat helpful
4 = It was quite helpful/I am quite satisfied
5 = It was very helpful/I am very satisfied

Degree of satisfaction with drug therapy among ninety-eight pathological blushing (PB) patients with or without associated hyperhidrosis. The patients were treated with 50–100 milligrams of sertraline per day.

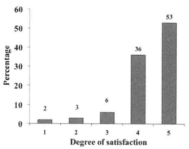

1 = I regret having had the operation
2 = It was not helpful at all
3 = It was somewhat helpful
4 = It was quite helpful/I am quite satisfied
5 = It was very helpful/I am very satisfied

Degree of satisfaction with ETS among 101 PB patients with or without associated hyperhidrosis. T2 or T2-T3 ETS were performed.

Index

Printed in Great Britain
by Amazon